Living
SKINNY
in
FAT
GENES

It's never too late to change your health outcome!

By applying simple principles and science to the realities of our everyday lives, we can modify our health risks, increase longevity and achieve better health.

You are what you eat!

Fat genes run in your family? Nobody in your family runs!

You only have one body, isn't it worth 30 minutes a day?

Felicia has been there—she's struggled with her own fat genes and has persevered!

Felicia speaks in her own voice, embracing the reader with her warm, friendly, and outgoing personality to set simple, realistic and attainable goals to achieve a healthier life!

Living SKINNY in FAT GENES

The Healthy Way to Lose Weight and Feel Great

Dr. Felicia D. Stoler, DCN, MS, RD, FACSM
Nutritionist & Exercise Physiologist

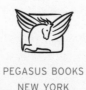

PEGASUS BOOKS
NEW YORK

LIVING SKINNY IN FAT GENES

Pegasus Books LLC
80 Broad Street, Fifth Floor
New York, NY 10005

First Pegasus Books trade paperback original edition December 2010

Interior design by Lorie Pagnozzi

Library of Congress Cataloging-in-Publication Data is available.

ISBN: 978-1-60598-116-1

10 9 8 7 8 6 5 4 3 2 1

Printed in the United States of America
Distributed by W. W. Norton & Company, Inc.

FOR ISABELLA AND ZACHARY

· ·

CONTENTS

You don't have to wear those fat genes your family passed down to you!

FOREWORD

∙∙

With all the research that has been done in the last 30 years about the human body, health, and disease… heart disease is still the #1 cause of death in the United States. Overweight and obesity, along with its comorbidites, are still on the rise… spreading across the globe… threatening the life span of humans… now impacting the children of the world (who may not outlive their parents because of overweight and obesity). Are we products of our environment or our genetic blueprint? If your family members are overweight or obese… are you doomed to the same outcome? The answer is no.

The information that consumers have been reading has not made a dent in changing their health outcomes. Misinformation, FADs (Fast Acting Diets), and generous interpretations of the science have only provided fuel to fire the confusion and aid in the yo-yo effects of "dieting" that many people have experienced. Americans have adopted an orthodoxy of food "beliefs" which are based on hearsay and anecdotal information, which has made it difficult to grasp the evidence-based science, which can ultimately impact their quality of life as they age.

In LIVING SKINNY IN FAT GENES™, I offer simple and realistic approaches to changing one's health outcome and improving your quality of life through behavior modification in nutrition, exercise, rest and time management. The only book of its kind written by a doctorally-trained, RD nutritionist, exercise physiologist, TV personality, journalist, and busy working mom of two, who can provide recommendations based on science and help you to apply the concepts to your life "habits" in a practical manner. For me, it's personal—as someone who struggled with my weight (along with bad "genes" handed down to me). After successfully overcoming a battle of the bulge, I made the decision to become an expert through formal education and training. I am uniquely positioned to share the secrets and solutions for living life in a healthful manner, while debunking the myths of diet, exercise, genomics and disease risk. I have been sought out by hundreds of media outlets over the last decade because I tell it like it is.

What I will share with you on these pages is based upon what researchers have observed over many decades, which I have used and incorporated into my private practice, speaking and personal use. Yes, I do practice what I preach… and so far, the results are there! Here's the best part—what you learn in this book is not that "diet" you go on and off of, but really this is meant to be a way of life. Your whole family can apply the principles in these pages. As a parent, I want my children to not only have a better life than me in all those "metaphorical ways"—but I really want them to have the gift of a healthy life, which comes from knowing that diseases can be prevented or even delayed. We know more about how our food choices and physical activity behaviors impact our bodies (from the inside out) than my parents' generation. My children have been my experiment in applying everything that I've learned about disease prevention and applying it to them since birth (really in utero). You are never too old to change your disease risk factors, but how will their health be from doing it early? Only time will tell.

The number of people to thank are so great—please don't be offended if I missed you. First, my darling children who have had to share their mommy with work, school and the world. Phillip, thank you for always believing in me. My parents, Francine and Jeffrey, have been my support my whole life, I am grateful that you have always been there to catch me. My brother Jeremy, my sister Suzanne (& Ivan) and her daughters—my nieces (Jessica, Sabrina & Olivia) who have learned to eat whatever they want in front of me. My aunts & uncles—I'm not cranky anymore. My late grandmother, Jeannette, who let me cook in her kitchen (my food is healthier) but was my larger than life role model for being a working mother, a leader, a volunteer and never was never was lean with the hugs and affection. My aunt Marilyn, who was like a second mother to me, who shared my passion for cooking and was my number one fan—I miss you so much. My oldest and dearest friends who have watched me "morph" into the person I am now: llene, Karen, David B, and AJ. My Tulane gals—Lisa, Gina & Paige. Sheren, Trish, Robert L, Evan, Julie G, Ann Y, both Carrie M's, Larry, Paul, Amanda, Dr. Aaron and Thasheda.

To my former nutritionist and exercise physiologist, Michele Vivas, who told me to stop listening to the muscle heads in the gym, throw out the diets from the magazines, eat some fat and let go.

I'd like to thank all of my graduate school professors, who are too numerous to name... but must thank Sharon Akabas, who made the notion of attending Columbia less intimidating and by giving me an opportunity to learn, so that I could leave my mark, by helping people to improve their health.

My dietetics colleagues Barbara Baron, Debbie Cohen, Tricia Davidson, the Nutrition Twins (Tammy & Lyssie), Kate Geegan, Mitzi Dulan, Heidi Skolnick, Robyn Flipse, Geri McKay, and Keith Ayoob. My ACSM colleagues—Lewis Maharam, Stephen Siegel, Neil Pire, Robert Sallis, Stephen Rice, Shawn Arent, and Stephen Perle. My professional cousin, Howell Wechsler.

My thanks to TLC & the BBC NY Productions for giving me the opportunity to host the second season of "Honey We're Killing the Kids!" I know the reality of reality television! I must thank all of my agents & their assistants—Babette Perry, Ira Stahlberger and everyone at IMG. My heartfelt appreciation and gratitude to Jennifer Unter, for believing in my message and working hard until we found the right publisher who would not make me compromise my ethics just to get a book! My gratitude to Jessica Case and Claiborne Hancock at Pegasus Books for making my wish come true. I thank all the individuals I have counseled and groups that I have spoken to—your input and questions are what help me to keep my finger on the pulse of what society perceives about this complex issue!

Most importantly—thank you for buying this book and taking the steps to learn how to Live Skinny in Fat Genes™ once and for all!

You only have one body, isn't it worth 30 minutes a day?

"Living Skinny if Fat Genes" . . . you just wish it could be so easy. Well, it is. As you read through the pages of this book I hope you will embrace my philosophy and recommendations along with tried and true advice that really works! I'd like to thank you for purchasing my book . . . Enjoy the journey!

Living SKINNY in FAT GENES

....

"If there is any deficiency in food or exercise the body will fall sick." —HIPPOCRATES

....

INTRODUCTION

From my experience, more people are concerned about how they look rather than their personal well-being. In LIVING SKINNY IN FAT GENES™ I will dispel the many myths that have been held as truths to so many of us. I hate the "D" word. To me, it is an acronym for "Did I Eat That?" This is not another "D" book about how to lose weight. This is a book about how to live a healthier lifestyle and in doing so the weight will come off. I promise you that.

LIVING SKINNY IN FAT GENES™ is a resource and tool to help you be the best that you can be and to maintain a healthy lifestyle so that you can enjoy a wonderful life. It's simple, realistic and attainable.

Why another book about diet, nutrition, exercise, and healthy living? Consider these questions: with over 5,000 books about nutrition, fitness, wellness and diets… why is obesity still on the rise? Why is there an increase in Type 2 diabetes? Why are cholesterol levels still elevated? Why is heart disease still the number one killer? Why are people still seeking out diet and nutrition advice? If we know that exercise improves health, why are we doing less of it? Nutrition and exercise intervention are the least expensive, least invasive and most effective ways to prevent and treat these diseases.

I am living proof that you can live skinny in your fat genes. As someone who went from always being at my "ideal body weight," feeling as though I woke up one day 25 pounds overweight, I was convinced that there was a mass growing inside my body because I could not figure out why I couldn't lose the weight. There were many people in my family who were overweight and obese. Did this mean my time was up and was joining the family fat gene pool? Working out twice a day, every day, learning as much as I could from the personal trainers at the gym, I read every article that I could get my hands on about exercise, weight loss and nutrition. I completely restricted my fat intake, ate strange food combinations, yet the scale was not going down…!

I went to a nutritionist and exercise physiologist in my mid-twenties. She helped me to dispel the myths and become more sensible about eating and exercise habits and behaviors. She told me, "Felicia, you're a smart girl, you read a lot, but you just don't understand the human body and how it functions in order to put it all together." Many people who read diet plans in books, magazines and on the Internet are in the same situation.

Crying in my nutritionist's office, I acknowledged that I was willing to trust what she was telling me was the *truth*. I had to relinquish *my* beliefs about nutrition and fitness and try to do what was suggested. It was worth giving up absolute control of information because I wanted to lose weight so desperately, to feel better, and live a long, healthy, and vibrant life.

So, how did I do it? Throwing away the "skinny" clothes, changing my food beliefs, making better food choices, watching portions, working out differently, incorporating rest into my routine and setting small, realistic and attainable goals. In addition I had to learn how to love "myself" no matter what size clothing I wore, no matter how much I weighed. I was not defined by my body—it was the person inside that mattered. After all, I was the only one who saw the numbers on the scale (scales are for fish, not for women), my body weight was not tattooed on my forehead, and gone were the days when clothing sizes were permanently displayed on the outside of jeans (thank goodness)!

The end result? I lost ten pounds over the summer and it took me over a year to lose the remainder… but I have kept it off ever since and lost all the weight after two pregnancies. Slow change was lasting change—but it was overall behavior that brought me back to my skinny jeans (okay—I had to buy new ones)!

It is essential for people to wear "blinders" and learn how to ignore most of the information that is clouding their beliefs and stopping them from losing weight. There are so many self-taught, self-proclaimed "gurus" of "flab." Everyone is an arm-chair quarterback (especially friends and family) when it comes to nutrition, weight and exercise. But do they all practice what they preach? I do. I knew that I needed to go back to school, to get the BEST education in order to truly have the foundation to be a nutritionist and exercise physiologist in order to help others. Nobody would want a doctor, dentist, nurse or psychologist to teach themselves their craft or skill. Nor would most want the hairdresser, mechanic, accountant, airline pilot or banker to be self-taught.

Why does this matter? Because people get what they pay for—plain and simple. Ask the "nutritionist" in the health food store for free advice and you get what you pay for. Does that individual understand the biochemistry and physiology of the human body? Nutrient metabolism? Was all personal health information disclosed to this person? If so, do they understand from a medical perspective your personal needs? Do they know about diabetes, high cholesterol or hypertension from a bio-physical perspective? Can they teach you how to integrate simple steps into your current habits and behaviors in order to help you achieve your health goals? Probably not. Within the pages of this book, I will provide the answers.

Now, ask any physician, how many courses (not lectures) they took in nutrition. Was it a full semester or a one-hour lecture? The answer will be surprising. Medical training in the United States does not require nutrition at all. Less than five percent of medical schools provide nutrition education to its students. How many chiropractors claim to offer nutritional counseling (what does that have to do with spinal alignment)? There are PhD psychologists who call themselves nutritionists, as do personal trainers. If you need quadruple bypass surgery— who do you go to? A cardiothoracic surgeon or a hypnotherapist? One wouldn't ask their dentist to treat acne, so why go to a professional who is not directly trained and educated in the appropriate field of specialty? It is amazing how many individuals want a piece of the weight-loss pie, without the education. Do people care how a celebrity lost weight? They write plenty of books, endorse all sorts of products. Do you know why? Because they are making a lot of money doing it; regardless of efficacy, it's about the almighty dollar, NOT your personal well-being. As Howard Stern used to say, "Who cares what celebrities think?" Caveat emptor—let the buyer beware!

Everyone wants a piece of the weight-loss business. The weight-loss industry brings in over $30 billion per year. It thrives on people failing at one technique and moving on to the next—what a form of job security! As one NYC endocrinologist so eloquently phrased it—these opportunistic people and companies proliferate quackery. Most of my clients have been so frustrated by the time they get to my office because they have tried "everything" else—with no long-term success.

With all the diet books and commercial weight-loss programs, why are we still an obese nation? Have our genes changed that significantly in the last half a century? The answer is "no." Natural selection and preferential survival genes take hundreds of years to evolve. The answer lies within a combination of factors—the society we live in, our daily lifestyles, along with the bombardment of chatter along the information superhighway. The science of nutrition, fitness and health is a relatively new science that is just that—SCIENCE. Yes, behavior modification is a vital, critical and essential component in weight loss and maintenance. However, the human body is a dynamic force, and as we learn more about its inner workings (from the body systems, to the cellular level down to the DNA), the better we can understand how to make changes to effect changes in order to live in a more healthful manner. Even if your genetic blueprint makes you predisposed to being overweight (like mine), you don't have to wear the fat genes that were handed down to you!

LIVING SKINNY IN FAT GENES™ will help you to understand how you can make simple, realistic and attainable changes to your everyday habits and behaviors as they relate to food choices and physical activity in order to reduce your body weight, reduce your risk for diseases associated with overweight and obesity, and live a healthier and happier life!

CHAPTER 1
Are Those Hand-Me-Down Genes?

• •

If your parents and siblings are overweight—are you doomed to the same fate? It's time to realize our roots and stop being slaves to our genes and our culture. Research has shown that for some of us, we are predisposed toward being more overweight than others. It is not just about excess body fat. There are people whose muscles tend to "bulk up" when they exercise (and you know who you are), and they sometimes appear to be overweight. Is your current body shape and weight due to your DNA alone? The answer is "no." The simple reason is the accumulation of your lifestyle habits and behaviors. It is never too late to change your health outcome or body shape. I am not suggesting that everyone work towards a "waiflike" image of oneself. For me, the notion of ever having bird-thin legs will just never happen because my bone and muscle blueprint has been set.

We have all evolved from humans who survived feast or famine. We have "thrifty" genes—which involve conservation of energy. So, having the ability to slow down one's metabolism when food (calories) are sparse and store fat when excess is available, makes our body the "bargain shopper." Do you look at your parents, aunts, uncles, grandparents, and siblings and wonder whose body yours resembles? You know, we are the product of our environment. In studies of twins who have been separated at birth and reared apart, genetics plays a role in resting metabolic rate; however, food consumption, sedentary behavior and physical activity are determined by the families' environment and learned behaviors. The twins who were overweight are those who were raised in adoptive families who were overweight. In other words, kids start to resemble their parents. There have been anectodotal stories of pets resembling their owners (yes, pet overweight and obesity is on the rise as well).

I will never forget one of my first private-practice clients… his food journal blew me away. On days one through four, he ate what I would consider two entrees—really huge portions at each of his meals. In one of his journal entries, he describes Sunday night dinner, "My mother makes meatballs the size of your head." By the fifth day of his journal, he ate visibly less food and left me a note on the bottom of the page that read, "Now I know why I'm such a fat f-ck."

It's a matter of what you get accustomed to. As I tell my own kids and children who come into my office, "You were not born with instruction manuals." Pediatricians, along with books and other resources, guide parents about how to feed children. However, there are other factors that influence choice: economics, cultural norms, parental personal preferences, other social inputs, availability, religion, food allergies, and intolerances.

I recently participated in a webinar for a company that claimed to have a genetic test to determine if a person has a particular gene, which would respond BEST to a particular type of diet AND specific type or exercise regimen. There were so many problems with the information provided—but the main challenge, as a practitioner, was this: what if an individual cannot or will not work out as recommended by this type of test nor willing to eat the recommended nutrient ratio? Can they not lose weight? The real answer is, that they can still lose weight. Test after test can tell us how our DNA may express itself, but it does not define our capability. Breast cancer screening for the BRCA (1 and 2) gene mutations is one example. Many women develop breast cancer without the BRCA mutations, and some women who have it, do not develop breast cancer. So what causes a mutation to occur or cells to start producing an undesired effect? The inputs from the environment can play a key role.

Epidemiology is the study of the relationships between disease, lifestyles and the environment. We often ask why something occurs and try to find a link between a cause and effect. This has been seen with diet and certain cancers, diabetes and heart disease. Many people assume that diabetes is caused by eating too much sugar, but it's a disease in which a person either does not produce adequate insulin to respond to blood sugar levels or their cells become resistant to insulin, which prevents blood glucose from being used for fuel in cells. It is a problem of "sugar absorption" inside the body on a cellular level, and while eating pure sugar doesn't help, it does not cause the disease.

The challenge is looking at an individual and the sum of their lifetime inputs. For example, a person recently asked me if açai is really a miracle fruit. My answer was, "For weight loss, no—there are no miracles. As a newly marketed fruit with high ORAC (oxygen radical absorbance capacity) values and potential health benefits—yes." However, assuming all other habits are good it might be of some nutrient value. So, if you smoke, eat a lot of fried food, consume excess calories, drink gallons of soft drinks and never exercise, well—one pill, potion or tincture will not be the cure-all for your health.

Do you eat to live or live to eat? My father's family lives to eat and they eat large quantities. It was not until my twenties that I realized that I could not eat the same quantities that I was accustomed to. I doubled my clothing size in a few years—I was 25 pounds heavier and really shocked as to how I got that way! What changed in my life was that I was working super long hours as a paralegal, NOT able to work out as often as I wanted to (this was before gyms had hours before 7 a.m. and after 9 p.m.). Eating high-fat food, drinking plenty of alcohol, and not sleeping enough were my culprits. The reality of my younger sister's wedding and getting into a size 8 dress from a 4 put me in a depressive state. After all the attempts at fad diets and excessive exercise yielded no significant results, I sought the advice of my physician. This was in the days when fen-phen was legal. I read all the literature about the potential side effects in his office and told him it was not worth the risk. I did want to lose the weight, though. He said he had just the gal for me. What I learned from her—which did help me to achieve my goal, I will share with you in these pages because I learned it in my training.

You can always buy off another rack!

CHAPTER 2
The History of Jeans (Food Consumption)

● ●

Just as blue jeans have evolved over several centuries, so have our eating habits. Jeans, or dungarees, were exported from India in the sixteenth century. This was a popular fabric for soldiers, which later was made in Europe. In the 1600s the raw materials for jeans came from Nîmes, France (de Nîmes—"denim"), and the dyed fabric was sold in the harbor of Genoa to soldiers (bleu de Gênes—"blue jeans"). The rest is for somebody else's book, but the point is, our present eating habits have developed over hundreds, if not thousands, of years.

We have all heard that we have evolved from cavemen who were hunters and gatherers. Food was scarce. Humans spent hours eating plants, berries and seeds—whatever they could easily get their hands on. Finding and killing an animal (or fish) was no easy task with primitive means. Until humans were able to harness the power of fire—all food was consumed raw. Nutrition knowledge did not exist; neither did food safety or sanitation for that matter. Humans ate for survival (just like other animals)… and many probably died from poisonous or contaminated food. There are some who theorize that fire changed the way humans lived and how our bodies changed through evolution to resemble our current design. This is part of what separated us from the animals and allowed our bodies to develop in a physiological way to adapt the digestive tract in a manner that was most efficient, while allowing our brains to enlarge to handle the expansion of intelligence. Those who were able to store and utilize fat effectively survived longer. Survival of the fittest is based upon genes, which may have really meant survival of the fattest.

Consider the crude weapons of ancient civilization: do you really think there was a lot of animal meat available for consumption? It was consume or be consumed. When animals were killed, entire groups and communities consumed the animal right away. Cooking was pretty simple—everything went in a pot, including vegetables and herbs. Our ancestors probably did not eat the variety we do now! Every part of the animal was used. Even their hides did not go to waste. Remember, there was no refrigeration to store the leftovers!

In addition, plant foods—leaves, berries, fruits, nuts and seeds—were consumed (these foods can't run away). Minimal food preparation occurred, if at all. People ate when food was available. An uncertainty about the food supply was the norm.

Hence survival of the fittest took on new meaning: feast or famine. Food was scarce. Over time, those who survived during periods of limited food availability were those who had extra fat on their bodies (the "designer genes").

Human metabolism is a self-preservation mechanism, slowing down, sparing precious fat stores, when calories are scarce. This will be discussed in more detail later in the book. Have you ever noticed the physiques of people who were the subjects of paintings, from previous centuries? Many were plump and cherubian. Wealthy people were fat people—they had the money to buy, prepare, and eat food. They had expensive genes. Being fat used to equate to health—at least when people weren't living past fifty. Assuming that among all people there are fat genes, have you ever seen a fat person emerge from a prisoner-of-war camp? Fat genes or not, those people look ghastly because they generally did not have access to adequate calories. Even in this century, in many African nations, women strive to be full-figured because the assumption is that if someone is thin, they have HIV/AIDS.

The agricultural revolution allowed humans to harness the power of Mother Nature to provide society with food in greater abundance. It was more than planting seeds and learning how plants grow. It included herding animals for food, which is part of every early religion's tradition and is mentioned in the Old Testament, the New Testament, and the Koran. Remember, there was no refrigeration until the twentieth century. Kosher and halal food rituals both have religious significance that may have evolved from the need to preserve food and prevent illness from food. One could argue that their methods of slaughter, food preparation (salting meats/fish) and avoidance of certain animals (pigs and scavengers) helped to reduce food-borne illnesses in a crude world.

While I was sitting in my chemistry class at Pace University (trying to fulfill my science requirements for graduate school), my instructor said something that has always stuck in my mind. When we were discussing carbohydrates and protein, she said she had come to America from the Caribbean because protein here is cheap. She went on to explain that protein of animal origin (bird, beast or fish) in the United States is very inexpensive, relative to its costs in other parts of the world. This was the first time I had heard this. As my education continued, I came to understand about access to food and supermarkets. In many low-income communities, access to fresh produce is scarce. The least expensive meats (which I will generally mean beef, poultry, and pork) were the fattiest cuts. The overall prices for food in these communities was higher.

If you look across cultures, and around the world, most dietary intake is predominantly plant-based. If you were to compare food recommendations of different cultures, the one thing they all have in common is the prevalence of grain products, fruits and vegetables, with animal-based products being consumed more sparingly—often as a flavoring ingredient versus the main focus of the meal. In most parts of the world, plant-based foods are more abundant, there is less risk of food-borne illnesses (although we have now been battling E. coli in produce due to inappropriate farming methods and unsafe handling after harvesting) and better storage capabilities (especially useful with limited resources and electricity), and it is more reasonably priced.

Where's the beef? Not in many parts of the world. Many Indians are vegans (strict vegetarians who consume no animal/fish products). In Asia, very few cattle are used for food. In Europe, with fears of mad cow disease, beef consumption has decreased. In the Americas, cattle is king! By no means am I making a statement against red meat. The truth is, I love all kinds of protein foods (even from animals), and this is entirely a personal decision that you must make for yourself. Far be it for me to turn down an opportunity to indulge in beef carpaccio, Parmigiano-Reggiano, fresh lemon juice, olive oil and arugula! Even with my family history of heart disease, I still enjoy eating steak periodicially.

I must also be upfront about dairy and milk products—I have been a spokesperson for the American Dairy Association, National Dairy Council, MilkPEP (Milk Processor and Education Program) and worked with Ovaltine and Nesquik. I think dairy products rock! There has been extensive research into the connection between dairy intake and weight loss. If you consider its protein content, milk is a very nutritious food. Humans have been drinking milk (human, cows, goats, and sheep) for centuries. Have you ever noticed that a lot of small children will not eat meat? It's because the taste is too strong and they don't like the texture. How can parents be sure that their rapidly growing child is getting adequate protein? Good choices for protein include fluid milk, yogurt and cheeses. Let's face it— humans have been consuming milk from animals for centuries; it dates back to herding cultures. Early civilizations learned that consuming milk from a cow, sheep or goat would yield more food energy, over time, to benefit more people, than by eating the flesh of the animal. This rationale is the same for eating the eggs of a chicken or hen instead of eating the whole bird.

What I want you to know is that any writer can self-select the data they want you to know, in order to validate their viewpoint. It can be difficult to be 100 percent objective if you have such strong convictions or opinions. My professional recommendations are gleaned from reading the various information, looking at what has been seen in history, and in practice. I have heard every argument against drinking milk, much of it based upon hearsay and myth. I believe in science-based recommendations. Some cultures—Asians and Africans—do not consume milk because they have a genetic predisposition towards lactose intolerance (you don't produce the enzyme lactase which is necessary to break down lactose). This is an example of a genetic trait that is passed down. So culturally, if most people in your community are lactose intolerant, most people would not consume dairy. After all, who would want to repeatedly eat foods that made them sick? Scandinavian, Italian, German, Russian, Mediterranean, Latino and French cuisines have relied heavily on dairy products. So people from different parts of the world have passed down distinct and unique genes to their offspring. We don't always like the genes that are handed down to us, but do not mistake lactose intolerance for a general statement that humans are not meant to consume dairy products! It is not based upon disease risk or hard evidence that humans should not consume dairy.

Even people who are lactose intolerant can consume some lactose/dairy. Yogurt contains cultures to help break down lactose, and many hard cheeses, such as parmesan, have low levels of lactose. We live in a time of food innovation, so products can be made without lactose or with Lactaid.™ Remember, all foods can fit—the key is to understand your individual needs. You already know your personal preferences. Humans can digest and absorb all types of foods. However, there are inborn errors in metabolism as well as malabsorptive diseases that can make this difficult for some individuals. I am about keeping to the scientific facts, not the hearsay or anecdotal evidence that keep the rumors and myths alive.

Do you have imported genes? With the exception of the First Nations peoples, we all do. There is a phenomenon called acculturation. When people immigrate, in this case to the United States, their genes do not change at the border per se, but their behaviors change as they take on the new ways of the society they have joined. So you see many people who arrived in the United States with a normal BMI (Body Mass Index) who, over time, become overweight or obese. Some people show up here and they plump up like a popover!

In every culture, eating—the gathering, cooking and consumption of food—brings people together. Whenever I'm in New York, I always ask taxi drivers where they are from, how long they have lived in the United States, and how they like the food here. During one of my many cab rides, a nice driver shared his story with me. He told me that he's gained weight since he's been in the United States. I asked him if he ate the same foods here that he ate back home. His answer was, "Oh no, I eat a lot of fast food and junk here but back home, lots of rice, roti and vegetables—not as much meat." My suggestion to him was to go back to eating the way he did in his native country.

Here is a brief description of typical foods in various cultures:

Northeast Asian—China, Japan, and Korea are known for grilling and frying in oil. Traditional foods include:
- Rice
- Garlic
- Fish (cooked or raw depending on where you live)
- Hot spices (chilies)
- Vegetables
- Ginger
- Noodles (rice, egg, wheat or potato based)

Southeast Asian—Cambodia, Indonesia, Malaysia, Singapore, Thailand, and Vietnam are known for their "light" and aromatic cooking, using such ingredients as:
- Citrus juices
- Herbs—basil, cilantro, lemongrass and mint
- Soy sauce
- Curries
- Coconut milk
- Ginger
- Noodles (rice, egg, wheat or potato-based)
- Rice
- Seafood
- Vegetables

Southwest Asian—Burma, India, Pakistan, and Sri Lanka have borrowed a number of Turkish foods. Some typical staples include:
- Nan (flatbreads)

- Kebab
- Mutton/Lamb
- Ghee (clarified butter)
- Hot peppers
- Cloves
- Curries
- Rice
- Chapati (made from wheat or barley)
- Yogurt
- Ginger
- Vegetables
- Legumes (lentils/chickpeas)

Latino integrates many various crops from around the Latin-American continent, including:
- Maize
- Beans
- Potatoes
- Nuts
- Vegetables
- Legumes
- Rice
- Quinoa (*KEEN*-wah)
- Yucca
- Tortillas
- Cheese
- Chilies
- Chicken, fish, eggs, beef, and lamb in small quantities

Caribbean food patterns have been influenced by the settlers in their region over the centuries and include Creole,

African, Indian, Hispanic, European and Chinese flavors. Main foods from this region include:

- Fruits—many exotic varieties: coconut, papaya, mango, plantain
- Vegetables—many exotic varieties—Yucca, sweet potatoes, tubers
- Curry
- Cinnamon
- Ginger
- Annatto
- Allspice
- Legumes (the largest source of protein)
- Goat, fish, chicken, pork
- Roti (flat bread)
- Cou-cou (cornmeal mush)
- Rice

Eastern European/Russian
- Grains: barley, wheat, oats, kasha, rye
- Breads
- Vegetables—many root vegetables, especially potatoes
- Fruits—mainly berries and non-citrus tree fruits
- Dairy—milk, cottage cheese, farmer cheese, yogurt
- Eggs, beef, pork, duck, chicken, lamb

Western European
- Fruits
- Vegetables—especially root vegetables, cabbage
- Herbs of all varieties
- Jams/jellies

- Grains—oatmeal, porridge
- Breads of all varieties
- Dairy—cheese, milk
- Eggs, beef, pork, chicken, fish, sausage, game
- Soups and stews

African
- Fruits—some wild varieties, watermelon, bananas, plantains
- Vegetable—cassava, yams, sweet potatoes, peas
- Nuts
- Seeds
- Dairy—milk, curds and whey
- Chilies
- Flatbreads
- Rice
- Cinnamon
- Cloves
- Stews
- Meat, poultry, fish—depends on the country. In many cultures animals are currency, and are used for their bi-products, not their meat. Since many Africans are Muslim, pork is not consumed.

Mediterranean
- Fruits
- Vegetables
- Grains—whole, bulgar, cracked wheat
- Couscous
- Pasta
- Polenta

- Dairy–yogurt, cheese, milk
- Legumes
- Nuts
- Seeds
- Fish, chicken, beef, lamb
- Olive oil
- Breads–pita

Persian/Lebanese/Egyptian
- Fruits–dates, figs, grapes
- Vegetables–peas, cucumbers
- Grains/breads
- Potatoes
- Beans/legumes–fava beans, chickpeas, lentils
- Tahini
- Nuts
- Seeds
- Small amounts of meat, fish, poultry, lamb
- Rice
- Pita
- Dairy–yogurt, cheese
- Mint, parsley, oregano, garlic, allspice, nutmeg, cinnamon
- Hummus
- Tabbouleh

In many cultures it is considered an insult to refuse to eat food that is offered. I have always found it entertaining when I have experienced people who are super picky with the foods they eat. In many parts of the world, food is scarce; respect for the hospitality that is provided is paramount, whereas in the United States, we often pick at or not eat food that is offered to us. In Africa, as soon as a guest arrives, food is provided—it is an insult NOT to provide it, and an even bigger insult NOT to consume it—even if one is NOT hungry. I know some of you are thinking, you never have a problem turning food down, right?

Asian foods typically are comprised of predominantly fruits, grains and vegetables, with smaller amounts of fish and meats added for flavor. Asian diets are lower in fat and protein overall, and the incidence of heart disease and cancer is less than in the United States. Certainly, there is more physical activity in Asian nations, fewer cars and even less public transportation. People are dependent upon their feet to get them places—even by bicycle.

Globalization of food patterns has increased the incidence around the world of chronic diseases that are typical in the United States, such as obesity, high cholesterol, high blood pressure, diabetes and heart disease. What is interesting to note is that these diseases used to be considered signs of aging, but they are now the result of certain lifestyle choices and are seen in many people under the age of fifty.

I am sharing this with you because if you take a good look at the eating habits across continents and cultures you will see that in most parts of the world the human diet has been predominantly plant-based: grains, fruits, vegetables, nuts, seeds and beans. In addition, dairy and eggs have been a source of protein, with other animal protein being consumed in much smaller quantities than they are in the United States. I am not saying become a vegan (and there is nothing wrong with eating vegetarian); what I am trying to point out is that many fad diets in the United States have been based upon the notion that we should be eating more protein and have demonized carbohydrates of all kinds. This has not been the case for health or longevity in other parts of the world or throughout history for that matter.

How have our eating habits contributed to our health care crisis? Well, as a nation it is no secret that we are larger than our parents and grandparents. In the United States alone, overweight and obesity are correlated with the leading causes of death and may decrease our lifespan by 5 to 20 years. The escalating costs of health care will have a direct impact on the government in regards to monies spent on research, treatment and prevention. On a national level, the Federal Trade Commission estimates that over $30 billion dollars is spent annually on weight loss products and services. The economic costs of an unhealthy diet and physical inactivity add up to almost $100 billion per year or approximately eight percent of the national health care budget in direct medical costs. The Centers for Disease Control reports that $31 billion (in year 2000 dollars) of direct treatment costs for cardiovascular disease was related to overweight and obesity.[*] It is not just about the financial strain on our country from the hard costs. It trickles down into sick days and other negative effects of disease. What is so sad about all of this is that it is preventable. We are not doomed—there

---

* Centers for Disease Control. Preventing Chronic Diseases: Investing Wisely in Health; 2005 (www.healthierus.gov/steps/summit/prevportfolio/PA-HHS.pdf).

is not a germ causing it, but we need to take some personal responsibility to help ourselves.

We have experienced the "supersizing" of our portions. One of my favorite illustrations of this is found on the National Heart Lung and Blood Institute Website (http://hp2010.nhlbihin.net/portion). There is a free PowerPoint that you can download that shows images of portions now versus 20 years ago AND the amount of exercise needed to make up for those calories:

20 Years Ago	Today	Calorie Differential	Exercise Needed
Coffee (with whole milk and sugar) **45 calories** 8 ounces	Mocha Coffee (with steamed whole milk and mocha syrup) **350 calories** 16 ounces	**305 calories**	**Walk 1 hour and 20 minutes*** *based on 130-pound person
Blueberry Muffin **210 calories** 1.5 ounces	Blueberry Muffin **500 calories** 5 ounces	**290 calories**	**Vacuum for 1.5 hours*** *based on 130-pound person

Another cause of our extra calorie load is the fact that many of us eat meals away from home. For some people, meals at home are pre-prepared and warmed up instead of being made from scratch. Cooking skills are no longer taught in many schools.

What happens is that you lose control over the calories and ingredients that are in your food when somebody else makes it. It can be very easy to finish an über portion at a restaurant if you are with others happily chatting away and all of you are eating similarly oversized meals. There are healthier options available at restaurants (see chapters 10 & 11), but many people do not choose their foods based upon what they need to eat, but what they want to eat or feel like eating at that moment.

We eat out of boredom and are bombarded by advertising reinforcing the reasons why we need to eat various food, drink different beverages and dine out at restaurants that have the resources to pay to capture your attention. Let's face it, in the United States, food is less expensive and many of us load up when there's a sale because we think it is a bargain- whether or not we need it!

There is also the perception that restaurant dining is less expensive and saves more time than cooking and eating at home. Cost can vary depending upon your ingredient choices, but certainly, there are less "healthier" options which are less expensive on most restaurant menus. There is a booming beverage industry providing sweet-tasting beverages (both no, low and high-cal) to meet our sweet tooth. When I was a child, soda was a treat and we had it a few times a month, NOT every day. While I'm a sports nutritionist who believes there is a value for sports beverages, they should not be consumed with meals, just to please our sweet tooth.

Our drive for sweet and salty foods can be modified. The more we consume them, the more we want (like certain addictive drugs). Likewise, if you decrease your intake of these flavors, your "drive" towards these will decrease. This is why I discourage even calorie-free, sweet-flavored beverages. It just whets one's appetite for even more sweets down the road. We can always change our tastes for food the way we change our taste for fashion!

So much of what I do involves listening to people—not dictating my edict or personal preferences, but understanding what habits they have, how they have evolved and how to modify current behaviors to bring about desired changes and results. It's that simple.

Let's talk about behaviors. I learned in graduate school and in many continuing-education lectures that it takes 21 days to change a behavior. Are behaviors simply a matter of will power? No, but it *is* about a choice. One patient told me that because he always watches television in the family room, which is adjacent to his kitchen, he CANNOT stop eating. He constantly goes into the kitchen to get more food to snack on until he's ready to go to sleep and then he's totally disgusted with himself. I know you are thinking: "Why can't he choose to stay put in front of the TV and not make trips to the pantry?" Well, habits are surprisingly hard to break and sometimes take a little something extra besides just willpower. We discussed options and as it turned out, his daughter was going away to college soon and so he decided to make her bedroom, upstairs and away from the kitchen, into a television room. Guess what happened? He stopped his constant grazing. This was not such a difficult thing to do and it was a simple way to help him to change his behavior. No pain, but lots to gain!

Behaviors are taught as well as learned. We acquire many of our behaviors during childhood; which is why childhood overweight and obesity is so alarming. Many parents treat their children the same way that *their* parents dealt with them. Essentially, hand-me-down behaviors. Now, we can choose to follow suit or change, modify or exclude behaviors (and deal with the consequences and repercussions accordingly).

Let's look at hunger, food and the body's need for calories! The human body is a pretty amazing and complex collection of systems that function and adapt to conditions. First, there is hunger… you wake up and your blood glucose (sugar) levels are low. You may feel sluggish and even have some hunger pangs (pains). As you start to *think* about food, your stomach and digestive tract may start to get revved up because the hypothalamus (your brain's control center) starts to release neurotransmitters to excite the receptors in your gastrointestinal tract. Gastric juices will be produced. Next, your sense of smell will further excite your brain in anticipation of the wonderful food that is about to touch your lips.

You know that feeling, when you smell something sweet and yummy baking or the aroma of French fries. The smell initiates the production of hydrochloric acid in your stomach; anxiously awaiting its mission to break down this magical food into smaller particles. This contributes to hunger pangs and the grumbling that we have all experienced at some point in time. So what happens after you eat? If you chew your food well, and don't devour your meal like it's an eating contest, you should become full.

FULLNESS & SATIETY [Suh-*TIE*-uh-tee]

Overfeeding begins in infancy—especially for those mothers who do not breast feed and are expected to feed their infant x number of ounces every set number of hours. If you watch infants carefully, they will turn their head away from food when they are done… however, the caregivers are conditioned to "finish the bottle."

For many people, their sense of fullness and satiety is a biofeedback system that will trigger our ability to STOP eating. However, there are others who genuinely lack the proper biochemical feedback mechanism to stop putting food in their mouths.

I have had patients with this exact problem… emotions aside, they genuinely NEVER feel full! For those people, learning appropriate portions sizes and knowing the number of servings they should eat each day, from each of the food groups, is critical. Keeping track of food is the only way to prevent excessive eating.

There is yet another group of people (and you know who you are) who emotionally eat. I actually lose my appetite when I'm stressed out, and though that is true for many people, for so many others, stress and anxiety are often satisfied, or at least temporarily relieved, when food or beverages are consumed. I know some people who cannot stop eating certain food because it "tastes so good"—they derive great pleasure from the tactile experience and flavor of the food on their tongue. The more they savor the flavor, the more difficult it can be to stop themselves! For some others, binge or overeating can be part of compulsive behaviors (as with ADHD) in which neurotransmitter levels do not properly signal the brain to stop. These people often eat until they are nauseous and incredibly uncomfortable.

It can be challenging to find some other activity or sensory stimulus to replace food. Some things you can do include drinking water, tea or coffee (without a lot of sugar), go for a walk, do some jumping jacks, squats, listen to soothing music or read a book! Also, while eating—slow down. Put your fork down between bites and chew your food well; then swallow.

CHAPTER 3
Designer Labels: Are All Threads (Foods) Created Equal?

∙∙∙

This chapter is going to zip up many of the food and nutrient questions that you have with regards to loosening the rivets on your food beliefs that have come out of marketing and science. At some point, you may have heard that body weight is all about energy balance: energy in (calories) versus energy out (physical activity)—this is true. This is the first basic premise of weight loss—there is no way around this (except if you fall into the category of folks who actually need to eat more calories each day to lose weight because you deprive your body of the amount of calories it needs for even basal metabolism). Before the TV show *The Biggest Loser* made its way into so many homes, Rena Wing, PhD at the Warren Alpert Medical School of Brown University and James O. Hill, PhD, at the University of Colorado Health Sciences Center established the National Weight Control Registry (www.nwcr.ws)—the original biggest losers. The database contains information on people over the age of eighteen who have lost 30 pounds or more and have kept it off for at least one year. Here is some important information about what they all have in common:

- 98 percent modified their food intake
- 94 percent increased their physical activity (walking being the exercise of choice for the majority)
- They don't skip meals, weigh themselves at least once a week, and exercise on average one hour every day.
- Most reported eating low-calorie (lower than what they ate before), low-fat diets with high levels of physical activity.

This is the stuff that registered dietitians (RDs) tell people all the time, but unfortunately, we live in a culture of quick results versus permanent solutions. So while this is the basic scientific principle of weight loss from a biophysical aspect, human emotion can be more powerful than our sense of doing what is best for our health, long-term weight loss, and maintenance.

The inherent premise of many commercial weight-loss programs includes some form of calorie restriction or set intake per day—but the formula is often based on some equation, but may not be as individualized as you would like. It's like going to into several clothing stores and knowing that you are one size in one store, like the GAP versus another size in a different store, like Ann Taylor. What you will learn is how to maximize your calorie "budget," so you will get the most "bang" for your calorie "buck"! This principle is called nutrient density. Essentially, how are you getting the most value (protein, carbohydrates, fat, vitamins, minerals and fiber) for the fewest calories. The reason is that by eating foods that have good components—"threads" if you will—you will be sure to put foods in your body that have some value to your body's basic needs.

Let's talk about FADs (Fast-Acting Diets). A FAD is any plan that (a) sounds too good to be true, (b) involves exclusion of a food group in whole or part, (c) claims that combining or keeping foods apart will increase weight loss or (d) claims to increase your metabolism. As you will learn, our bodies can pretty much digest any and all foods—in any combination and at any time of the day. We need nutrients from every food group and that is a fact. You are about to learn why this is true.

Speaking of which, let's just get a quick nutrition 101, which I explain to all my clients. The human body is absolutely amazing. From the moment we think about foods, smell, see and taste it—our body gets ready to digest it. You know what food looks like going in—and we all know what it looks like after our bodies have broken it down and extracted all the essential nutrients from it. Digestion begins in the mouth—when we chew our food (called mastication) into smaller pieces. What we are doing is lubricating our food with saliva, which contains enzymes that begin to break down starches. I know people who inhale their food—and you would think it goes down whole… but remember, your mother probably said to chew your food well. There is a body of research that looks at the benefits of chewing your food finely (the number of times you bite down before swallowing) and weight. There are lots of reasons to consider this. First, because the more time you take to eat your food, the greater the likelihood would be that you would not overeat because it would take you longer to finish your meal and give your stomach time to send a message to your brain to STOP eating. Another basic reason would be the amount of calories that are expended by your jaw and tongue in the grinding process (so basically, increasing your "physical activity" level while eating). Finally, by taking the time to break down solid food in your mouth into smaller particles, it can be digested a little easier by your body, with less feelings of something lying like a brick in your tummy.

Moving down the chute—once the food is in your stomach, it is acid-washed to break it down into even smaller particles and blended into a mixture we fondly call chyme. From a satiety perspective, when you eat a meal with protein, fat and fiber, it slows down the rate at which foods leave your stomach and make their way into your small intestines for absorption. How does your stomach NOT get a hole from the low (acidic) pH? Well, it's considered a mucous membrane, so it is protected from its own cannibalistic actions!

The next stop is the small intestine, via the pyloric sphincter (or valve) where, like a car wash, your gallbladder and pancreas blast this moist mixture with bile, bicarbonate and other digestive enzymes, through the pancreatic and bile ducts in order to neutralize it and make it ready for the big break down. Understand that all food, on a chemical* level, ultimately is made up of one of three macronutrients: carbohydrates (sugar/ glucose), protein (amino acids) or fat (fatty acids). It doesn't matter what form it came in as—this is how the body identifies it and responds to breaking it down and absorbing the nutrients through the lining of the small intestine and sending off, via the portal vein, to the liver for some filtration before making it available to the body. Vitamins and minerals are also removed from particles (just as you would pull a tag off your clothes) and absorbed along the way.

Carbohydrates are pretty much the main component of all plant-based foods: grains, vegetables, fruits, nuts, beans and seeds. The only place carbohydrate is found from an animal source is in milk. It is the master fuel that the body uses

---

* In this instance, the word chemical is used to imply chemistry and the molecular makeup of food versus something synthetic.

for energy. We can only store around six hours' worth of fuel from carbohydrates. We have limited capacity for long-term storage. In our bloodstream, carbohydrates become blood glucose. It can be stored in muscles and in the liver as glycogen. In the absence of carbohydrates from our diet, our bodies will break down protein (muscle mass), use the amino acids and combine them with fatty acids to make glucose. This is an expensive way to make the fuel we need, but this is how our bodies function. On another note, when we are using this mechanism for fuel, it creates ketones in the blood and urine. Ketones cause a decrease in blood pH, making it more acidic. This is NOT a desired "normal" state (although some high-protein diet books would tell you otherwise). When ketones become more concentrated in the body, it can cause coma and death.

Protein is used for muscle tissue. It is the main component in blood (hemoglobin) and is necessary for our immune system to function properly. Ultimately, protein is broken down into its smallest units: amino acids (which are the building blocks of protein). A very small amount of amino acids are used for fuel. Protein comes from the muscle of animals: poultry, cattle, sheep, goats, wild game, fowl, and fish. Protein is also found in eggs and milk. When found in a plant source, it is not necessarily "complete": nuts, seeds, vegetables, legumes, and grains. What makes a protein "complete" is whether it has all the amino acids. There are twenty different amino acids, nine considered "essential"—those that cannot be synthesized (created) at all by the body or cannot be synthesized in amounts sufficient to meet physiological need. Here's an easy way to remember them: TV TILL PM H: Threonine, Valine, Tryptophan, Isoleucine, Leucine, Lysine, Phenylalanine, Methionine, Histidine. Leucine, Isoleucine and Valine are the amino acids that may spare protein degradation. The nonessential amino acids are those that the body can synthesize or create in the body and are Tyrosine, Leucine, Arginine, Alanine, Aspartate, Cysteine, Glutamate, Glutamine, Glycine, Proline, Serine, and Asparagine. Protein is stored in muscle tissues—and this also has a fixed storage capacity.

Fat helps to transport and store fat-soluble vitamins, maintain body temperature, provides fuel and serves as a master storage for excess fuel (like a supersized walk-in closet). Fat is found in the fat of animals, under the skin, marbleized in the muscle, in dairy, nuts, seeds, certain plants which we derive oils from: olive, avocado, coconut, corn, soy, nuts and seeds.

Fiber is an interesting substance. It is found strictly in carbohydrates or plant-origin foods (unless it's been added or fortified in foods). The simplest explanation is that the fiber found in plants provides the basic structure for the plant, like the threads in your jeans. Think of the strands you find in celery or the opaque coating around each kernel of corn. There are two different types of fiber: insoluble and soluble (think of it as polyester versus cotton).

Here's a chart comparing insoluble and soluble fiber:

	Insoluble Fiber	Soluble Fiber
Function	• Controls pH and acidity • Moves bulk though the intestines	• Slows down the emptying of stomach contents (affects satiety and glycemic uptake rate) • Binds with fatty acids (helping to lower cholesterol)
Benefit	• Prevents constipation by increasing transit time of waste (including removal of toxins) • Helps prevent colon cancer by quickly removing toxins from the large intestine while maintaining optimal pH	• Helps regulate blood sugar levels in diabetics • Lowers total cholesterol and LDL cholesterol (bad cholesterol) reducing the risk for heart disease
Food Source	• Skins of root vegetables and fruits • Nuts • Seeds • Green leafy vegetables and green beans • Wheat • Corn • Oat Bran	• Beans and legumes • Oats/oat bran • Fruits • Vegetables • Flax seed • Barley • Nuts • Psyllium husk • Barley

Why am I telling you this? As the tag line reads for the clothing chain Syms, "An educated consumer is our best customer." So when you read or hear information with regard to food, you too can now be an educated consumer. In the past, I taught an introductory nutrition and health course, and this basic information about human nutrition can empower students, even after half a semester, to have all the ammunition they need to debunk many food and diet myths by understanding the basic science of how our bodies use food and what foods are comprised of.

The simplest explanation is that your liver and blood stream does not care how a carbohydrate entered your mouth: as a slice of bread, a teaspoon of sugar or a stalk of broccoli. It all gets broken down into its simplest units (monosaccharides: glucose, fructose, galactose). Without getting into too much detail, all monosaccharides or sugar molecules cannot leave your liver as anything other than glucose—period. This is the master fuel for your body. Your brain relies exclusively on glucose for fuel.

Speaking of which, let's look at the metabolic activity and percent energy expenditure of your basal (resting) metabolic rate of your organs[*]:

Liver	Brain	Other Organs	Skeletal Muscle	Kidneys	Heart
21%	20%	20%	22%	8%	9%

So, as you can see, your brain requires a good amount of fuel to keep it functioning properly.

---

[*] **Human Nutrition and Dietetics**, 10th ed. J. S. Garrow, Ann Ralph, William Philip Trehearne, James A. Ralph. Elsevier, 2000, p. 40.

CHANGING FASHION

Just as jeans have gone from baggy to tight, high-waisted to low-waisted, food recommendations have changed. Do you remember hearing that butter was bad for you? Do you still think you can't eat eggs if you have high cholesterol? Eat fish because of the essential fatty acids? Don't eat fish because of the contaminants? Eat fat-free, sugar-free, carb-free? What is a person supposed to do?

Science is a learning process. The science of nutrition and health has changed or modified our recommendations based upon what we have learned or observed. It is the interpretation of cause and effect. The same has been seen with prescription and over-the-counter medications. As time passes we find out something may no longer bring about the result it was thought to OR our testing methods have become more sophisticated, so we can measure markers in a new or different manner.

When the media rush to report a new finding, take it with a grain of salt (even though we all need to cut back on our sodium intake). As I have learned in graduate school, one study is just that—one study. In order for the findings to be relevant and acceptable, the study needs to be reproduced and repeated many times to yield the same results in order for us to draw real conclusions. It's like knock-offs in fashion—can you make something that appears identical?

DESIGNER FRUITS AND VEGGIES—ARE THEY REALLY PREMIUM THREADS?

Did you know that the word "superfruit" was first used as a

marketing term in the food and beverage industry in 2005? You have seen these names—some you may be unsure how to pronounce (or spell): açai, blueberries, cranberry, goji, grapes, guarana, mangosteen, noni, pomegranate, and sometimes coconut are perceived to have magical health benefits! Some of these are grown domestically—while the remainder are imported from all over the world. It is all about the marketing and perceived benefit. Just like your designer jeans—is the denim from Levi's that much different from the Gap or Diesel?

Style matters, but in this case, it is a matter of a manufacturer or processor creating a demand by implying some health benefit. Each one, when consumed in mass quantity, allegedly has the magic to undo all the accumulated "damage" that your less-than-perfect food intake and not-always-consistent exercise have done to your body over your lifetime! Well, they certainly are great fruits and juices and can be healthy additions to your diet, but they are not "stain removers." Nor does consuming concentrated levels of these fruits (or the elixirs explained later in this chapter) dry clean your DNA or reverse heart disease, cancer or diabetes. Marketing and advertising puts the notion in our minds that we need to seek a product out—people are paid good money to do this. Remember—buyer beware. Just because you see something in print that makes a claim that the research is supported by science, unless you have the head to look up the original research and read it yourself (which I could never have comprehended properly before graduate school), does not mean it's true. There is plenty of misinformation in the media, and to an untrained eye, a good advertorial is difficult to distinguish from a legitimate piece of scientific literature.

As a whole, eating a variety of fruits of many different colors and textures has its benefits because of the unique pigmentation (color) of the fruits, which we refer to as phytonutrients or phytochemicals. The more colorful your plate, the more nutrient-rich your meal. Variety is the spice of life, and the same should be true of the food you eat.

ORGANIC THREADS

As a registered dietitian, I have been asked many times if I eat organic foods. My answer is yes, but I don't go out of my way to buy them. While I would agree eating organic would better, it is not always what is best. Here is my logic: I look at the big picture—beyond my food budget. Yes, we can be food elitists and suggest that everyone eat organic food. First of all, the cost can be prohibitively expensive. Second, organic standards are not the same around the globe, so essentially, you don't know if your food is really organic in the way you think it should be. Third, what is the carbon footprint of getting the food to you? This is a determination of the cost of transporting and storing the food until you purchase it—which can be VERY expensive (not to mention the effect on the environment to get the food to you). Fourth, the actual vitamin and mineral content of organic foods is not significantly different from nonorganic foods—if at all. Fifth, organic does not ensure food safety in handling, storage, packaging and shipping foods. Finally, just because it's organic does not mean it's healthy.

At Teacher's College, I learned from Dr. Joan Gussow—the mother of the nutritional ecology movement—that it is far better to eat seasonal, regional foods. What that means is buying and consuming foods that have been grown close to your home. Why? Because once land becomes homes, buildings or parking lots, the likelihood of that land being used to grow food is slim to none. I live in New Jersey—known as the Garden State—in an area where there are still many farms. Green spaces are not only good from an aesthetic standpoint, the plants recycle carbon dioxide and produce oxygen, and can provide fruits and vegetables, and serve as fodder for animals for human consumption, which is a good thing! In addition, we should not rely on imported foods. This does not imply stifling international trade, but, if we cannot create our own food in our own country, we will be dependent on those who provide it to us—much as we are for fossil fuels. As we have seen in changing climates, there are times where extremes in weather—heat or frost, lack of rain, insect or germ infestation—can wipe out entire crops and leave regions barren and its foods inedible. Take the rising cost of fuel: it has impacted food costs on many levels. If we grew more food near our homes, the price of transporting and storing the foods would be less and would help to lower our costs.

As for the bigger issue of antibiotics, growth hormones and pesticides, I appreciate the concerns from a health viewpoint. However, there are not as many antibiotics and growth hormones used in animals as are rumored—nor are measurable traces showing up in what you eat. The pesticides that are used in plants are there to keep the insects and germs out of your produce. There would be plenty of fruits and vegetables left on supermarket shelves if they were laden with holes, if the colors were not deep and leaves crisp or appeared moldy. We know to wash produce, and there have been no links to serious diseases as a result of pesticides used in our plant foods. Could it be that we just aren't eating enough fruits and vegetables overall? The pollutants in the air we breathe are probably worse than the trace amounts of pesticides we might consume. The likelihood is that in the course of your life you will consume foods that have not been produced using the organic method. So essentially, you are potentially being exposed to these alleged substances. It is very difficult to control, and at the end of the day, is it going to improve your life, your health or your life expectancy? Pick your battles. For you, right now, it's weight and health.

Indeed, organic farming methods are much better for the environment, and in many instances organic produce can withstand extremes in weather conditions compared to their non-organic counterparts. Labor costs are higher on organic farming and the process of organic certification can take quite some time and be expensive. These costs are passed along to all of us. If you have a limited amount of resources to spend on food, are you really going to pay two to three times more for an item? This is reality. Have you ever met a farmer near you? I have met many; as a group, they will tell you how difficult farming is—not only in labor but in making a living. Farming has not been the most profitable industry to be in. The good news is that people have a newfound interest in small farms, and their numbers are on the rise. Even I have had the idyllic fantasy of owning a farm—but then the economic variables have dissuaded me from earning my living from the land. What I recommend—which is what I do—is to support your local farmers. I go to local farm stands from May through October to get my produce. In the grocery stores near your home, try to select locally grown produce. The same is true for dairy products—especially milk. Try to get milk that comes from local dairy farms.

Another thing you might try is growing your own food. Start with herbs and vegetables like tomatoes, squash, green beans and cucumbers and see what you can achieve. It can be easy and rewarding to eat what you produce. Personally, I find weeding a garden rather cathartic—in addition to it being really solid exercise. If you don't have outdoor space to grow anything, try taking it indoors. Many herbs can be grown indoors in small pots. I have used an Aerogarden™, which is a hydroponic system for homes, to grow salad greens and herbs. Super easy to use and fun for me and my children.

So does the place where you purchase your food mean it's healthier? Is organic food healthier for you? These are among my favorite myths. A patient once told me that she only shops in Whole Foods and was shocked when I told her that not EVERYTHING in the store is necessarily GOOD for you. After all, they do sell fried snack chips and plenty of energy-dense yummies that even I have a hard time rationalizing which food group it may fall under (love My Pyramid's "discretionary calories"). She would be much better off stocking up on lean proteins, whole grains, fruits and veggies at any supermarket than a tub of ice cream from the Whole Foods. I do shop in Whole Foods occasionally, because they carry several brands and products that I cannot find elsewhere.

PROMISES TO MAKE YOU LOOK SKINNY IN YOUR JEANS—MAGICAL ELIXERS ARE NOT THE MIRACLE STAIN REMOVER!

Super juices, anything that offers a detox, cleanse or will melt away the fat (like a candle) are definitely making false promises. Did you ever notice how many of these miracle products are sold through multilevel marketing (MLM) programs? I am not saying that the success of MLMs is not worthy of a good MBA's case study for the success of marketing, sales and distribution. However, I am saying that just because thousands of people consume it does not mean it works. These products offer the world: enable us to lose weight, provide more energy and alertness, clean our insides out (as if our body is a toilet that needs flushing), and—my favorite—may cure an ailment. For the number of times I have been offered opportunities to get into one of these MLM opportunities—whether it was for health or beauty products—I have yet to meet one of those folks who really became a millionaire selling this stuff! Besides, my personal and professional goal has been to help people live a healthier life and to fight obesity. Making money doesn't prove my success—you do. Just to reinforce this hole in your jeans—it is about behavior modification: diet and exercise.

SUPER FOODS

Designer fruits, berries and veggies—are their health claims true? Why are these magical potions only available through multilevel marketing "schemes"? Can any foods really burn fat? Wishful thinking, but no. There are foods that can be beneficial in reversing and reducing the risk for heart disease (again, the #1 killer in the US) and some cancers. I remember learning about these super foods while in graduate school. These are still the top foods for health:

- Almonds
- Apricots
- Avocado
- Broccoli
- Cantaloupe
- Carrots
- Flax seed
- Garlic
- Grapes
- Green peas
- Green Tea
- Olive Oil
- Onions
- Oranges
- Red pepper
- Soy
- Spinach
- Strawberries
- Tangerines
- Tomatoes

- Wheat germ
- Whole grains
- Wine or purple grape juice (like Welch's)

What these foods have in common are unique protective nutrients that can alter health over time. They are nutritionally sound, offering an array of essential nutrients, reasonably priced, accessible throughout the year, and are adaptable to any cuisine. So, while there are new plants with pigments and nutrients being discovered, the same ones are still out there helping our bodies to be healthy and ward off disease.

Avocados

When I went to college, I was blessed to have a best friend from Dallas, Texas, and she taught me how to cut and eat an avocado (thanks, Lisa). I remember the creamy texture, and it was a delicious to eat with tortilla chips. I came home and was making guacamole at my parents' home all the time! I remember hearing around that same time too that avocados were "fattening." In graduate school, I learned that avocados have "good fats"—mono- and polyunsaturated fatty acids. In addition, they are loaded with vitamins and minerals— making them as good as a multivitamin! They have 20 vitamins, minerals and phytonutrients—including vitamins E, C, folate, lutein, beta carotene, iron, potassium, and fiber to boot! They act as a "nutrient booster" by enabling the uptake of fat-soluble vitamins. A common misperception is that they contain cholesterol. Avocados contain beta sitosterol, a plant sterol, which can help to lower cholesterol. In addition to eating cubes or slices of avocados, I have always liked to mash it up and use it as a spread on bread and sandwiches (in lieu of mayonnaise). My pediatrician recommended it as an early food for my daughter. She would gobble the avocado cubes—and so would I!

Flax Seed

You may have heard a lot about this funny little seed—which is brown, golden or yellow in color. I keep a stash of ground flax seed in my home and add it to everything: pancakes, cereal, salads, yogurt, tomato sauce, and stews. It is an excellent source of ALA (pre-cursor to omega 3 fatty acids found in fish oil) and lignans (benefit the heart and may have anti-cancer properties). It can help to reduce serum cholesterol, and contains B vitamins, calcium, iron, magnesium, phosphorous, potassium, and zinc. Added bonus—it's a good source of fiber! Sometimes I enjoy whole flax seed—but from a nutritional standpoint, the best way to reap the benefits is to consume it ground.

Almonds

I have always loved raw almonds purely for the taste and ease of measuring (super easy to count out 24 for an ounce). When I figured out they were a great food to ward off hunger pangs between meals or before a party to prevent pigging out when I arrive, I let all my clients know. I went for a presentation by my colleague Dr. Michelle Wien about almonds and their amazing health benefits. When her talk was over, I pulled my little plastic bag of almonds out of my pocketbook. She has worked with the Almond Board of California. On their website (www.almondboard.com) they sell a tin, the size of an Altoids tin, to put your serving of almonds in! They are an excellent source of protein, magnesium, and potassium. When consumed with a meal, almonds can decrease the surge in blood glucose afterwards. There are heart-healthy benefits, including cholesterol-lowering effects (LDLs are lowered by the monounsaturated fats) and decreased risk of heart disease from antioxidant vitamin E.

The flavonoids found in almond skins team up with the vitamin E found in their meat to more than double the antioxidant punch either delivers when consumed separately. Twenty potent antioxidant flavonoids have been identified in almond skins, some of which are well known as major contributors to the health benefits derived from other foods, such as the catechins found in green tea, and naringenin, which is found in grapefruit. Manganese, copper and riboflavin are all found in almonds and help with energy production. Alpha-tocopherol (vitamin E) may help neutralize nasty free radicals that can damage your cells, tissues, and even your DNA. A one-ounce serving of almonds contains a similar amount of total polyphenols as one cup of green tea and ½ cup of steamed broccoli. While many people forgo nuts because of their calorie content, consuming nuts regularly can help to prevent weight gain. One ounce of almonds provides 3.5 g fiber, which helps fill you up and prevents you from being hungry for less nutrient-rich snacks later.

Apricots

Fresh apricots are an excellent source of vitamins A, C, E, potassium, and iron, as well as a great source of beta-carotene.

I'm a big fan of dried apricots because they have even greater concentrations of these nutrients and are so portable! Apricots contain nutrients such as vitamin A that promote good vision. Vitamin A, a powerful antioxidant, quenches free radical damage to cells and tissues. Free radical damage can injure the eyes' lenses. The high beta-carotene content of apricots makes them important heart-health foods. Beta-carotene helps protect LDL cholesterol from oxidation, which may help prevent heart disease.

Apricots are a good source of fiber, which has a wealth of benefits, including preventing constipation and digestive conditions such as diverticulosis. Most Americans get less than 10 grams of fiber per day. A healthy, whole-foods diet should include apricots as a delicious way to add to your fiber intake.

Quinoa (*KEEN*-wah)

Quinoa is an ancient grain that is making a comeback in a big way. It is great hot or cold! Quinoa is high in protein (balanced set of essential amino acids), fiber, phosphorous, magnesium (responsible for relaxing the body's blood vessels and the production and transport of energy), riboflavin (facilitates energy production in cells), iron and copper. It is gluten free and easy to digest. Quinoa will absorb the flavor of anything you cook it with or add it to!

Don't know a good brand of assorted mixed whole grains? One of my very favorites is Kashi 7 Whole Grain Pilaf. You can eat it hot (like oatmeal or rice) or cold. When I cook it, I like to add dried cranberries for added flavor. It contains whole oats, brown rice, rye, hard red winter wheat, triticale, buckwheat, barley, and sesame seeds); one half cup cooked has 6 g fiber and 6 g protein.

THE MAIN BENEFITS OF WHOLE GRAINS

The benefits of whole grains most documented by repeated studies include stroke risk reduced by 30 to 36 percent, type 2 diabetes risk reduced by 21 to 30 percent, heart disease risk reduced by 25 to 28 percent, and better weight maintenance. Still not convinced? Other benefits indicated by recent studies include reduced risk of asthma, healthier carotid arteries, reduction of inflammatory disease risk, lower risk of colorectal cancer, healthier blood pressure levels, and less gum disease and tooth loss!

Assorted Threads

There are many whole grains on the list, and luckily they have become much easier to find in mainstream supermarkets:

- Amaranth
- Barley
- Buckwheat
- Corn, including whole cornmeal and popcorn
- Millet
- Oats, including oatmeal
- Quinoa
- Rice, both brown rice and colored rice
- Rye
- Sorghum (also called milo)
- Teff
- Triticale

- Wheat, including varieties such as spelt, emmer, farro, einkorn, kamut, durum, and forms such as bulgur, cracked wheat and wheat berries
- Wild rice

Studies show that eating whole grains instead of refined grains lowers the risk of many chronic diseases. While benefits are most pronounced for those consuming at least 3 servings daily, some studies show reduced risks from as little as one serving daily. The message: every whole grain in your diet helps!

Dark Chocolate

You know this is the only reason to eat chocolate, right? Just kidding. Who said healthy foods can't taste good? Dark chocolate contains flavonoids, which act as antioxidants, and can help to reduce blood pressure. It may be good for your heart and help to lower LDL cholesterol. Dark chocolate stimulates endorphins, which provide feelings of pleasure (just like shopping, right?). It contains serotonin, which acts as an antidepressant, and contains theobromine, caffeine and other substances, which are stimulants.

Buckwheat (a.k.a. Kasha)

Buckwheat groats are the hulled grains of buckwheat; they are nutritious but hard to chew, so they are often soaked and cooked. Buckwheat/soba noodles are popular in Asian cuisine. Buckwheat can be made into pancakes and is also in farina—which is a breakfast food (porridge). Buckwheat contains no gluten, so people with celiac disease may consume it, but, it can be a food allergen by itself. Tolerability varies by individual.

Beans

Now we can regress to childhood. Beans are good for your heart, although the more you eat, the greater the likelihood that you will fart—which is okay! Beans are rich in fiber and protein. They contain calcium, potassium, vitamin B6, magnesium, folate, and alpha-linolenic acid. Beans help to curb hunger and may reduce a person's risk of developing diabetes, heart disease, cancer, and obesity. Beans have beneficial phytochemicals as well as antioxidant properties. In general, darker-colored beans, such as red and black, have stronger antioxidant properties. Beans are a type of legume, which also includes foods such as peas and lentils. Generally, one half cup of any type of legume has roughly the same amount of protein as an ounce of meat.

Nuts

Nuts are rich in protein, fiber, antioxidants (vitamin E & selenium), plant sterols, and mono- and polyunsaturated fats (omega-3). There is an approved FDA health claim for almonds, hazelnuts, peanuts, pecans, pine nuts, pistachios and walnuts. Scientific evidence suggests but does not prove that eating 1.5 ounces per day of most nuts as part of a diet low in saturated fat and cholesterol may reduce the risk of heart disease.

Pomegranates

When I was a kid, my grandfather called them a "Chinese apple," and it was a treat for him to bring me one from a Lower

East Side market in Manhattan. Pomegranates are rich in calcium, potassium, folate, vitamins K and C, phytosterols and beta carotene. They have very high antioxidant properties (they contain tannins, ellagic acids and anthocyanins) and are commonly consumed as juice. Pomegranates may be useful to prevent LDL (so-called "bad") cholesterol from oxidizing, to improve the amount of oxygen getting to the heart muscle of patients with coronary heart disease, and to delay the development of certain tumors.

Benefits of Omega-3 Fatty Acids (fish oil)

Fish oil contains essential fatty acids, which are important for cell production and renewal. It can support good mood and improved blood circulation and is recommended by the American Heart Association. There are two omega-3 fatty acids: eicosapentaenoic (EPA) and docosahexaenoic (DHA). Fish oil has been shown to be supportive in the prevention of cardiovascular disease, cancer, arthritis, respiratory conditions and neurological disorders, including bipolar disorder and depression. It's a heart pleaser—it lowers blood triglyceride levels, reduces the risk of heart attack, reduces the risk of dangerous abnormal heart rhythms, reduces the risk of stroke, slows the buildup of atherosclerotic plaque, and lowers blood pressure. Fish oil reduces stiffness and joint tenderness associated with rheumatoid arthritis. Unfortunately, we may not be able to consume adequate levels from fish alone, so taking a supplement can be an asset.

There are lots of cool foods to eat, to help you Live Skinny in Fat Genes™, and they taste good, too! So think about adding some of these foods to your weekly regimen for added health and weight-loss benefits!

CHAPTER 4
Stretch Denim? You Are What You Eat

• •

If I eat fat, will I be fat? If I consume large amounts of protein, will I gain muscle mass and lose weight? These are among the myths to be riveted off your jeans! Does muscle turn into fat when it's not being used? You are setting yourself up for weight-loss failure if you go on a crash diet, skip meals or think that if you eat food after 8 p.m., it will remain in your stomach until you wake up the next day (or go directly to your inseams)!

Research does show that diet composition may resemble our body composition. Where does exercise come into play? We need to learn how to eat foods in a manner that helps us to achieve our goals. Are all vegetarians healthier and leaner?

Nope, and many are crapatarians at best! Where are carbs in our diet? Just about everywhere. Do carbs turn into fat and land directly in our back pockets or in those saddle bags? No.

In some cultures, people still eat only one meal a day. However, research shows that eating small frequent meals will help you to keep your metabolism revved up, and you will feel so much better, too! I have always recommended consuming three meals and three snacks because it keeps your blood sugar at a level to prevent fatigue and keeping your gastrointestinal tract working out (the thermic effect of feeding).

HOW DO YOUR PANTS FEEL?

Your gluteus maximus muscle does not turn into a fat pad. If you don't work out, your muscles may get smaller. We call it the use-it-or-lose-it principle when it comes to muscle mass. And while a pound of fat weighs the same as a pound of muscle (hint—a pound is a pound is a pound), when you exercise and are trying to lose weight, sometimes the numbers on the scale increase—temporarily, because your muscles are getting bigger. This is a good thing because it will increase your metabolism (which means that at rest you will burn more fat for fuel), and it will decrease the circumference of your limbs (this is where toning comes in). Fat stores do not get toned, they increase or decrease. Your muscles do the toning and hopefully you will use up those fat stores. You will find that your energy level, strength and stamina improve! As an added FYI: the muscles in your legs are the largest muscles in the body. Keep this in mind when you are planning your physical activity strategy.

FAT-FREE EATING

As a practitioner, the only time I really see fat restrictions in people's diets is when there is an eating disorder involved. We *do* need to eat fats because they are an essential nutrient, just like less-maligned vitamins and minerals. Eating appropriate amounts of fat will not make us fat. Remember, they are necessary for transporting fat-soluble vitamins into our bodies. Fat is usually added to many foods in the cooking process. If you dine out at a restaurant and want to know if they are using fat when they cook your meal, by all means—ask! You pay for it, you have a right to know. I get asked, Isn't bread or pasta fattening? The answer is that any calories that you eat in excess of your daily needs can be fattening. So eating a big loaf of Italian bread or a pound of pasta in one sitting is not what I would consider portion control (we'll get to that later). However, those foods, as they are made, are not fattening. What you put on them, however, has the potential to blow the calories and fat content through the roof.

DO CARBS TURN TO FAT?

This is one of the most frequently asked questions. It's like asking if cotton denim turns to polyester in the wash. In the body, carbohydrates circulate as blood glucose and are stored as glycogen. They do not get stored in fat cells. However, if we have excess calories in our diet and we are not utilizing fat for fuel, then more fat will be tucked away for storage. People who watch me eat (trust me, even my friends are curious to see what I eat to stay skinny) are often shocked at the volume of carbohydrates that I eat every day. No kidding. I eat lots of carbs every day. It really is my secret to skinny. From the starchy variety to the fruits and veggies—I have seldom found a carb I did not like!

WHAT IS PROTEIN, ITS ROLE IN THE BODY, AND WHY IS IT IMPORTANT FOR OVERALL HEALTH?

Protein comes from the Greek work *proteios* (of prime importance). It is vital for our body and is important for the growth and maintenance of body tissues: lean muscle tissues, heart muscle, and the gastrointestinal tract. Amino acids are the building blocks of protein and are part of hormones (thyroid, insulin, glucagon), enzymes, antibodies, and energy. Protein is important in the bloodstream for transportation of nutrients, blood clotting, and maintenance of fluid, electrolyte, and pH balances. Protein must be available at all times to build protein for new tissues and to replace worn-out cells. People think that if they exercise, they put extreme wear and tear on their muscles, but the cells that turn over the most frequently are those that line your gastrointestinal tract (every three days!).

The body does not have a storage form for protein to be used as energy the way we do for carbohydrates (glycogen) and fat. So the body must dismantle its tissue proteins from blood and liver, then from muscles and other organs. Even pro athletes know that this is the primary reason why we do *not* encourage athletes to refrain from eating carbohydrates, because in the absence of adequate "fuel" the body incurs wasting of lean body tissue. Our goal is NOT to decrease or slow down our metabolism!

DO YOU NEED MORE PROTEIN IF YOU ARE WORKING OUT?

People who exercise vigorously every day may need more protein than a sedentary person, but it is probably not as much as you think. The recommendations are based on nitrogen balance. What makes an amino acid molecule unique is a nitrogen atom. Nitrogen balance is the amount of nitrogen consumed compared with the amount excreted in a given time period.

- The RDA is 0.8 grams/kg of body weight per day.
- Endurance athletes need 1.2-1.4 g/kg of body weight per day.
- Strength athletes need 1.4-1.8 g/kg of body weight per day.

You can look at your daily protein intake needs in terms of specific numbers (grams/day) or in terms of percentage of calories. Since most people do not have access to all the food labels for items consumed, and to decrease obsessive behavior, I find it more realistic to consider protein needs as the percent of daily caloric needs: 20 percent from protein, 50 percent from carbohydrates and 30 percent from fats (the good ones). Most Americans tend to consume more than adequate quantities of protein. I think of it as one or two small servings a day of protein, which can include poultry, meat, fish, nuts, beans, eggs, or soy (tofu). Personally, I am a flexitarian—I skew vegetarian with small amounts of animal protein in my diet.

You may be concerned about the timing of your protein with

regards to your day. The chances are pretty good that you will probably get a little bit of protein every time you eat. It is important for bioavailability for the body for use internally and not for fuel. It takes longer to digest, absorb and utilize protein than carbohydrates, which are digested right away. I often find it funny when someone suggests a protein bar for energy before exercising, because other than making you feel full, it may not provide you with the fuel you need to get through your workout!

WHAT ARE THE BEST FOOD SOURCES FOR PROTEIN?

All types of protein from animal sources are more concentrated in amino acids and are considered "complete" with all essential amino acids, and can be digested and absorbed with great efficiency. Certainly, I always encourage consumption of whole foods when possible. Legumes are plants of the bean and pea family that contain nitrogen in the plant's seeds, which are rich in protein compared with other plant foods and are 80 percent digested and absorbed. Grains and other plant foods vary from 60 to 90 percent. Cooking in moist heat improves denaturation (breakdown for digestion), whereas dry heat can impair it. Think about beans—could you imagine eating a dry pinto bean? However, after being soaked in water and cooked, it is easier to digest. Dairy products are also an excellent source of protein.

CAN VEGETARIANS GET ENOUGH PROTEIN?

Vegetarians can get adequate quantities of protein from non-animal food sources. Remember, when someone says they are a vegetarian, there is not one assumption about the foods that they will or will not consume. For this purpose, let's consider a vegan, someone who will not consume any foods that came from an animal. We just discussed complete proteins. Incomplete proteins are proteins lacking, or low in, one or more of the essential amino acids. How do you make a complete protein? Combine foods from two or more of these categories to obtain complete proteins:

- Grains
- Barley, bulgur, cornmeal, oats, pasta, rice, whole-grain breads
- Legumes
- Dried beans, dried lentils, dried peas, peanuts, soy products
- Seeds and nuts
- Cashews, nut butters, other nuts, sesame seeds, sunflower seeds, walnuts
- Vegetables
- Broccoli, leafy greens, other vegetables

CRAPATARIANS

While this term is not in Wikipedia yet, I started using it while working on my doctorate. I was analyzing the food journals of my fellow nutrition graduate students. A few were also in the animal science department (at Rutgers) and said they were "vegetarians." Well, they may not have wanted to eat animal foods for various reasons, but I'll tell you, they had very little regard for the foods they put into their bodies! The colors of the rainbow did not come from fruits or vegetables, but from candy.

(Last I checked, Skittles don't contain phytonutrients.) Snack chips were consumed in lieu of veggies, and plenty of other "junk" food replaced nutrient-dense ingredients. Ultimately, there were lacking many, many essential nutrients!

What about protein bars, shakes & supplements? Will they give me more energy for working out?

Ask sports nutritionists about supplements and they should ask you, "What is it that you hope to achieve or replace in a bar, shake or supplement?" To athletes, the word "energy" means fuel for exercise. However, many bars and shakes that are high in protein and low in carbohydrates are going to give one satiety and perceived energy, but not necessarily energy in the metabolic sort of way. Certainly, there are times when all of us have been eating on the run, and keeping a bar handy for an emergency pick-me-up in lieu of fast food is a good thing. I do not recommend eating bars instead of food as meal replacements. They just do not give you the overall satisfaction and feelings of fullness as eating a meal. If you are in a pinch, that is one thing, but in place of a balanced meal, it is not the best choice!

What types of protein supplements (if any) are best?

Consider starting with whole foods. Can you add nuts, nut butters and seeds to your diet? How about dairy products? I'm a big fan of tuna or salmon packets—they make great grab 'n go snacks. Hard-boiled eggs and cooked edamame are also very portable. Again, I always urge you to chew your food and select foods that resemble their form in nature!

Supplements—Patches on Jeans

Do you think that there's a miraculous product out there that can improve your workout performance, give you more energy and build your muscles faster? Well, before I give away the ending to the story, let's consider what you may have heard from friends, on the Internet or seen at a health food store or gym. Many consumers believe that dietary supplements and herbs are regulated by the government to ensure that the products contain what they claim, are safe and effective, and that any advertising related to these products are true. There is an important set of rules out there called "DSHEA," which stands for Dietary Supplement Health Education Act of 1994. They protect the supplement industry—not you. Here's what you need to know: DSHEA does not require supplements to be proven safe or effective before they are marketed and sold. So, essentially, you are the guinea pig for the manufacturers.

You may have heard of a product called ephedra. Many people died from using ephedra before it was banned. As one of my graduate professors, Dr. Ronald De Meersman, said, "There's no such thing as a free lunch." What does that mean? Simply, there is no miracle pill or potion out there that can replace good eating, exercise and plenty of rest to improve chances of losing weight and keeping it off without a potential for harm. Is your desire to lose weight worth dying for? We would all agree that it is not. Even super-low-calorie diets can cause death. Even though you may be struggling with your weight, enjoy life! Being happy and having a positive outlook can help you to get into those skinny jeans!

Let's consider the various types of supplements on the

market. Some provide hydration (fluids), others provide fuel (carbohydrates, fat and possibly protein), others claim to provide energy (we'll get to that), and finally, some claim to have mystical powers to alter your body's chemistry and possibly increase your muscle mass!

Why would I consider a supplement that claims to increase energy bad? When anyone asks me about ways to increase energy, I ask, "What do you mean by energy?" To a sports nutritionist, energy means fuel (carbohydrates, protein and fat). To me, it sometimes means making sure you are getting adequate sleep. However, in the supplement industry, energy is an added boost or edge that is not necessarily able to be documented or proven.

Caffeine is an ingredient found in chocolate, soda, coffee and some teas. However, it is also added to some beverages, bars, gels and pills to give people more "energy." Caffeine is a stimulant that increases your heart rate and can make you feel more alert. It also has a diuretic effect (it increases urination). A little bit of caffeine can be safe, but too much can be harmful. One of the goals during working out is to improve your performance so you can accomplish the same work load with a decreased heart rate, which occurs from training adaptation. So why would you try to increase your heart rate? Need I say more? Okay, I'll just add that too much caffeine will keep you up at night, preventing one of the other mantras for you: getting enough rest!

Some supplements claim to change the way the body's

hormone and energy systems normally work. They are substances that claim to build muscle, mimic anabolic steroids, increase human growth hormones, suppress your appetite, add naturally occurring substrates to your system [individual amino acids (glutamine, taurine, glycine) or compounds like creatine or chromium piccolinate], or provide excessive levels of vitamins and/or minerals. Finally, beware of the sales pitch "the product is *all-natural.*" Just because a substance is naturally occurring does not make it safe. You may have heard that Americans have the most expensive urine in the world!

Use of products may create what is called the "placebo effect"—in that your mind may play a powerful role in your perception that the supplement may have improved your performance. Is it really just mind over matter? Where can you go for more information? The Food and Drug Administration Center for Food Safety and Applied Nutrition website (www.fda.gov/Food/default.htm). Remember to eat well, drink fluids, watch your portions and exercise to lose weight the old-fashioned way! Do you think these jeans ever go out of style?

I'll tell you a story about going to a small health food store where I asked the salesperson, "What is the most popular item you sell?" She responded that it was the protein powders because they help people to bulk up and gain muscle mass. She also added that it was important to drink water and that without the water, the muscles would go away. I did NOT tell her what I do for a living, but I did feel like an investigative reporter. I asked her what the mechanism of action was to cause this to occur and she said, "I don't know—that is what I was told to say." The people who sell these products care about making money, not your health!

Exercise, rest and eating a balanced diet are the best way to increase muscle mass and boost your metabolism. The other important aspect to consider is your genes because we all have a genetic predisposition for a maximum amount of muscle mass that we can attain naturally. Basically, once you reach your maximum growth potential, the only way to bypass your DNA is to use substances that are considered illegal and dangerous (e.g., steroids and growth hormones). The reward is not worth the risk. Ask any former bodybuilder who has had health problems as they age. Those jeans are in serious need of repair from all the wear, tear and abuse!

CHAPTER 5
Can You Wear (Eat) White?

∙ ∙

Welcome to the world that fights so hard for equality of people regardless of skin color—yet we have gurus telling us that eating "white" foods are bad for us. In the United States, we have fought for racial equality for decades, so now we have turned our discrimination on foods by color (or the lack thereof). Have you ever heard of something so ridiculous? Do you think that once your genes touch down on U.S. soil that white foods will kill us? When we compare traditional diets from across the globe that had been healthy in the past, we see that white foods are the staple of most diets. In Asia, there is an abundance of white rice. In Africa, Europe, and many Mediterranean diets, white-colored flour (even though it comes from wheat) is used to make croissants, baguettes, pasta, pita, roti/

chapatti and even tortillas. Pastas from rice and wheat are consumed everywhere else in the world without guilt.

I once got in a heated discussion with another nutritionist about brown rice being better for you than white rice. I took out two boxes and compared them. The difference was that there was one tiny gram of fiber in the brown rice versus no fiber in the white rice. Guess what? Rice is not a good source of fiber… not worth offending a friend at a dinner party or battling with your kids about eating it.

I got an interesting phone call from the father of a high school athlete who was going to decide if I was "worthy" of working with his son based upon how I answered the question "Is it okay to eat white bread?" I told him that the color didn't matter as much as the fiber content. I explained that some brands of white bread have fiber while some brands of whole wheat bread may not have much—it all comes down to the number of grams. Well, he didn't like that answer and insisted that the color of the grain made all the difference. It comes down to science, and the science has not demonstrated any real health difference. As far as I know, once food starts to be digested and broken down into smaller particles, once it gets to the liver, all carbohydrates, regardless of origin, cannot leave the liver as anything other than glucose. As one of my professors at Rutgers said, "Carbohydrates keep your brain happy." I know I need to keep my brain well-fed or I can't work!

WHOLE GRAINS VS. WHITE BREAD

White bread is made from wheat flour that has been stripped of its bran and germ and has been bleached. This process does extend the shelf life of white bread, but it also renders the flour with little nutrient value. Fortification is now mandated, to add thiamin, riboflavin, niacin, folic acid and iron back into flour products.

Whole grains, or foods made from them, contain all the essential parts and naturally occurring nutrients of the entire grain seed. Even if the grain has been processed (e.g., cracked, crushed, rolled, extruded, and/or cooked), the food product should still deliver approximately the same rich balance of nutrients found in the original grain seed.

As of now, the problem that I have with food marketing is that we are placing a strong emphasis on the words "whole grain," yet there is no measurable amount we can recommend to people and it is not labeled to quantify its volume per serving. So, a more important part of the food label to read is really the grams of fiber per serving. Let's keep it simple for you. Aim for at least 4 grams of fiber per serving—independent of food color!

I love some of the pastas available in the supermarket today—my favorite being Barilla Plus. It looks like "white pasta" but it's loaded with fiber, protein and essential fatty acids. My children figured out a long time ago that I was trying to get them to eat "healthy foods." Whole wheat pasta was spit out time and time again. I chew down just about anything, but have found that if the harsh food critics that are my children like a "healthy food"—then even my picky clients would probably like it, too! So the simple answer is yes you can eat white foods without worrying about people snickering because you are wearing white jeans before Memorial Day or after Labor Day.

Cravings

I sometimes have cravings to go shopping for new clothes, but it seldom is indicative of a lack of items in my closet that I can wear. Craving, by definition is an intense, urgent, or abnormal desire or longing. How about food cravings? You know the feeling. You hear, or see, or smell, or sometimes simply think about a particular food or substance, and you *must have* it —now. At some point, all of us have experienced this feeling. As ubiquitous as food cravings are, it is far from clear what exactly they are and why they happen. And these uncertainties can help us ascertain how to respond to a craving. Here's what we do know and how it can help you the next time you feel a strong, specific, food-related urge.

The body does not necessarily crave what it needs nutritionally. The occasional exception is sugar (glucose), for which we may feel an overwhelming desire for sweets when blood sugar levels are low. This feeling is more often indicative of overall hunger than of a need for something intensely sweet. The solution is clear—eat or drink something (just about anything will do) to boost that sagging blood glucose. You may crave salty foods during heavy workouts and/or in warm weather, when the loss of electrolytes in sweat may be greater than at other times.

Most other cravings seem to be as much psychological as they are physical. A craving can be a desire for something other than calories. For most of us, food engages all the senses— taste, smell, touch, sight, even sound. This explains how we can walk into a restaurant not feeling particularly hungry, and yet start salivating when we catch a whiff of roasting meat. Or see a snack food commercial while watching TV late at night—again, not feeling terribly hungry—and suddenly develop a case of the munchies. One of the reasons so many people crave chocolate is its creamy, rich texture and mouth feel. Others crave the crunch of potato chips or the frosty coolness of ice cream. Personally, I am a savory snacker, but do not get between my mouth and chocolate when I am PMS-ing! Though the response to a food's sensory properties is biological, we know that you might salivate, and your stomach may even rumble, and yet the cause may not necessarily be hunger-based. Rather, you want the food in question because of the many other ways in which it will satisfy your senses.

Research supports the relationship between mood and food. I have had many patients over the years who are emotional eaters. If you are one, you know what I'm talking about. Sometimes we relieve stress when we eat a comfort food (which varies by individual). In one study reported in the journal *Appetite*, carbohydrate cravers felt distressed before their craving, and relaxed and happy after satisfying it. Protein cravers were anxious and hungry before satisfying their craving, and happy and energetic after eating the foods they desired. Cravings tend not to be triggered by sudden, acute bouts of stress, such as being cut off by a car in traffic, but rather by chronic anxiety or tension—ongoing issues at work, trouble in a relationship, or the like. For many, cravings strike in the late afternoon or evening, when we tend to relax and unwind.

Many people's cravings are satisfied by what we call "comfort" foods. Often these are things we consumed in childhood or at other happy times in the past—chocolate cake, ice cream sandwiches, mashed potatoes, macaroni and cheese, and the like. Often these yearnings may relate to a desire to return to a time when we were nurtured and protected.

Get a handle on your cravings

Here's where all foods can fit. I suggest that you can satisfy a craving with a small amount of the desired item rather than attempting to resist the urge. Since cravings are usually not about hunger and deprivation, this strategy should cause the craving to dissipate. Attempting to ignore a craving can backfire because the yearning only grows to the point where satisfying it may result in overconsumption of the food in question. In other words, have a few Hershey's Kisses now rather than downing an entire pint of premium double-chocolate ice cream in four hours!

While watching your weight, you may want to try to distract yourself from a craving, because sometimes when you are on a weight-loss regimen, you may feel restricted in some way, which increases your desire for a food you may feel is a "no-no." We have become conditioned to assume that being on a DIET (yes, I used that word) means that you need to sacrifice something— which turns out to be a food or beverage you may start to crave. I suggest starting with a tall glass of water and wait to see if the urge passes. If it does pass, you may have just been dehydrated and not realized it. Exercise can be your ally here; try taking a short run or walk, doing some yoga, or even stretching for five to 10 minutes. The craving may well pass. If it doesn't, follow the advice above and yield to it with a modest serving of the food in question.

If your cravings seem stress-induced, it makes sense to work toward a resolution of issues that are causing conflict. If you're unable to do this on your own, you may want to use the services of a psychotherapist. Certain foods may trigger cravings so predictably that you're best off keeping the foods at arm's length. For example, I don't allow Cheez Doodles in my house, workplace, or car because I know if they're close at hand that I'd crave (and eat) far more of them than is good for me. I swear they call to me from my pantry, "Eat me, Felicia, I'm here." Avoid markets or restaurants that sell or serve foods that may trigger your cravings.

Managing your cravings

While cravings are normal and some may be unavoidable, there are ways of reducing their likelihood and frequency. Here are some strategies:

- Limit your intake of sugar substitutes and increase carbohydrates, especially high-fiber foods. In my experience as a dietitian and nutritionist, I have seen many clients control their sugar cravings by making these two changes. When you eliminate or restrict your carbohydrate intake, your body seeks revenge in the form of extreme sweet cravings!

- Eat a variety of foods on a regular basis to make sure you are meeting all your nutritional needs. Don't exclude food groups from your diet. Eating plans that restrict consumption of certain food categories—carbohydrates, for example—can trigger cravings for those foods, sometimes even leading to binges.

- Try different food textures, tastes, and aromas. Varying the sensations associated with food adds to the overall pleasure of eating, which can reduce cravings. Eating mushy or soft food gets boring and does little to stimulate your mouth cavity!

- Eat spicy foods because they fire up your metabolism and are so intensely flavorful it's tough to eat them in excess.

- Eat small, frequent meals—for example, breakfast, lunch, and dinner with a morning, afternoon, and evening snack—to maintain stable blood sugar levels. Don't wait until you're ravenously hungry before you eat or you may make poor food choices or overeat. If you stay up late, have a small snack before bedtime, especially if you exercise first thing in the morning.

- Drink plenty of water. Full hydration helps regulate blood glucose, preventing dips in blood sugar, while dehydration can mimic the symptoms of hunger.

- Eat slowly; it takes about 20 minutes for the brain to receive the message that the stomach is full.

- Get enough sleep. Lack of sleep can increase the body's levels of stress hormones, and high levels may trigger cravings.

- Moderate your caffeine and alcohol intake. Too much of either of these substances can cause blood sugar levels to fluctuate, potentially triggering cravings. Also, it decreases the likelihood of your getting the drunken munchies!

- Do you tend to crave something sweet after a meal or late at night? To avoid post-meal and between-meal cravings, include a salad or side dish of vegetables, some soup, or an extra serving of rice or pasta with your meal. If you do get hungry later, have some fruit or other healthy alternative to a traditional sweet dessert (see box for suggestions).

Angel Food Cake (with or without fruit)

Fruit & yogurt parfait with cereal or granola

Skinny Cow ice cream

Graham crackers

chocolate-covered/dusted almonds

chocolate-covered pretzels

Jell-O fat-free pudding (not sugar-free)

Fruit smoothie

As a health-minded person, you've probably read a million articles about what, when, and how much to eat and drink. You may think there's little new information and advice out there for you. However, what is tried and true can help you to LIVE SKINNY IN FAT GENES™.

CHAPTER 6
Off the Rack: Sizing (Portions & Calories)

So you are probably wondering—does one size fit all? Well, of course not. Your genes do not inherently tell each of us how many calories to eat each day (or how much exercise to do). The basic formula of energy balance is key. If you gorge yourself on luscious energy dense foods in excess of what your body's needs are… then you will find some extra junk in your trunk!

SIZING CHART

When determining your health goal, remember to make your goals attainable. Start with small changes; maybe modify one or two things in your life. If it's weight, look at changes in ten percent increments. What does that mean? Look at the height and weight chart below.

RULE OF THUMB FOR IDEAL BODY WEIGHT

Ft./Inches	Women			Men		
	Low	Medium	High	Low	Medium	High
4'9"	73	85	94	80	88	97
4'10"	81	90	99	88	94	103
4'11"	87	95	105	90	100	110
5'	90	100	110	95	106	117
5'1"	96	105	116	101	112	123
5'2"	99	110	121	106	118	130
5'3"	104	115	127	112	124	137
5'4"	108	120	132	117	130	143
5'5"	113	125	138	122	136	150
5'6"	117	130	143	128	142	157
5'7"	122	135	149	133	148	163
5'8"	126	140	154	139	154	170
5'9"	131	145	160	144	160	177
5'10"	135	150	165	149	166	183
5'11"	140	155	171	155	172	190
6'	144	160	176	160	178	197
6'1"	149	165	182	166	184	203
6'2"	153	170	187	171	190	210
6'3"	158	175	193	176	196	217
6'4"	162	180	198	182	202	223
6'5"	169	185	204	187	208	230
6'6"	171	190	209	193	214	235
6'7"	176	195	215	198	220	242
6'8"	180	200	220	203	226	249
6'9"				209	232	255

For example, a 5'4" woman weighs 175 pounds and she wants to lose 43 pounds. What is a realistic goal? She can aim for an initial weight loss of 17.5 pounds, and when she gets to 157.5 pounds, she will reassess. Her next goal would be a weight loss of 15.7 pounds—which would bring her to 141.8 pounds. In order to reach her goal of 132 pounds, her intermediate weight loss is less than 10 percent of her goal.

Let's start with how to determine your body's caloric needs. It begins with something called your basal metabolism, which is the sum of all calories (or energy) it takes for your body to operate while at rest. This includes your heart, brain, kidneys, liver, lungs, etc. Then there is the amount of calories you burn while you move (fidgeters burn more calories). There are many calculators that you can find online to help you to determine your metabolic rate AND keep track of calories used throughout the day.

CALCULATING ENERGY NEEDS

In order to determine your goal, you need to have an action plan with regard to your calories consumed. Here is the equation you need to know:

Energy Balance = Energy Consumed (calories)−Energy Expended (exercise)

If you want to lose weight, you need to take in fewer calories and expend more energy in the form of exercise. If you want to gain weight, you must consume more calories (but do not give up exercise) than you need. Use the Harris-Benedict Equation (HBE) for calculating your caloric *need*. The formula does have its limitations for people who are very muscular and for those who are morbidly obese. Remember, this is an estimate, not an absolute number. There needs to be starting point—and this is how we get there. You may also use the HBE calculator on www.bmi-calculator.net/bmr-calculator/harris-benedict-equation/.

FEMALES

661 + (4.38 x weight in pounds) + (4.38 x height in inches)–(4.7 x age) x activity allowance "aa" (see below) = caloric need

Now complete for yourself

(remember to do those calculations in the parenthesis first):

661 + (4.38 x_____weight in pounds) + (4.38 x_____height in inches)–(4.7 x_____age) x_____activity allowance (see below) = caloric need

661 + (_____) + (_____)–(_____) x_____ aa =
_____ caloric need per day

MALES

67 + (6.24 x weight in pounds) + (12.7 x height in inches)–(6.9 x age) x activity allowance "aa" (see below) = caloric need

Now complete for yourself

(remember to do those calculations in the parenthesis first):

67 + (6.24 x_____weight in pounds) + (12.7 x_____height in inches)–(6.9 x_____age) x_____activity allowance (see below) = caloric need

67 + (_____) + (_____)–(_____) x_____ aa =
_____ caloric need per day

Activity Allowance—when determining your activity allowance, remember that because you are BUSY does not mean you are physically active!

- 1.15 HBE—Sedentary
- 1.3 HBE—Light Activity (normal daily activities)
- 1.4 HBE—Moderate (exercise 3-4 times per week)
- 1.6 HBE—Very Active
  (exercise more than 4 times per week)
- 1.8 HBE—Extremely Active (daily exercise and a job
  that may include manual labor)

Since your goal is weight loss, you need to create a calorie deficit. Safe weight loss can be achieved at a rate of one half to two pounds per week. At some point, you may plateau in your weight loss, so that could mean, in some instances, eating more calories! Exercise is in essential part of this process for building muscle mass (and increasing your metabolism) instead of simply increasing fat stores!

To lose this amount of weight each week	Eat this many fewer calories
1/2 pound	250 calories
1 pound	500 calories
1 1/2 pounds	750 calories
2 pounds	1,000 calories

Example:

Your calculated need for intake is 3,000 calories per day, and you want to lose weight, slowly, so you would start by consuming 3,000 calories −500 calories for weight loss = 2,500 calories per day. In addition to a reduction in calories (or intake), you should also increase your physical activity each day!

Why do you need to know this value? Because we do not intuitively know how many calories we need to eat each day. Our genes did not come with the care label sewn inside. We have had to rely on decades' worth of research to understand why some of us are heavier than others. In some situations, our genes may be to blame because the amount of lean muscle mass that we can maximally achieve naturally has been predetermined in our thread count (muscle fibers).

I've had people come into my private practice and tell me how many diets they've been on and how they need to eat less than 1,200 calories a day in order to lose weight. So I ask, if they know that, then why are they coming to see me? The truth is that unless you are vertically challenged (your jeans are "floods" instead of long), you really need to eat at least 1,200 calories, if not more, a day. Let's face it, 1,200 calories is not a lot of food. You might lose weight on it, but you may kill somebody in the process because your hunger will be voracious (jean envy) with an equally bad mood to go along with it.

Does the size matter? Well, when the calories are counted at the end of the day, then yes—size does count! We all want to fit in smaller jeans, right? So you need to eat smaller amounts— plain and simple. This is where the fun begins! This plan is not about eliminating food groups, making you walk around with a scale or measuring cups. Let's face it, we don't have calculators on our tongues. What I do with my private-practice patients is show my clients how, for the most part, they CAN enjoy most of the foods they like to eat, as long as they can get enough servings from each of the food groups. By working within their current habits and behaviors, we create meal plans that are sensible and integrate individual preferences, which is why they are more likely to stick to their meal plan and be successful in their goals! By the end of this book, you'll know how to do this for yourself. This is how you end up with a plan that is custom-fit for you!

CHAPTER 7
Putting Your Genes on the Spin Cycle: Exercise

• •

I kid around with my friends: I say that if I didn't have to work, or if I had the financial resources that many celebrities have, I would be at the gym or working out for at least two hours a day. I sincerely mean it. It's not about body weight as much as making my body strong and feeling good. Exercise gives off endorphins that can give you a natural "high." It can also help to relieve stress—which is important for both mental AND physical health. The American College of Sports Medicine along with the American Medical Association and the President's Council on Physical Fitness recently dubbed May *Exercise is Medicine*™ *Month*. The reason is that if exercise came in a pill and doctors prescribed it, people would take it. Research shows that exercise is an essential nutrient for our brains to grow, and it makes us feel better and have more energy!

How many times have I been asked about how to lose weight without exercising? All the time! How did we become a society of overstarched duds? We are too stiff to move; our sitting around causes our bodies' aches and pains. The thought of exerting energy can be fatiguing before we even get out of bed each morning. I don't expect everyone to become a gym rat, and to that end, I actually prefer the term physical activity to exercise when working with people who have not been athletic in the past. Why? Well, it's less intimidating, and as I will show you, by increasing your physical activity throughout the day, you will find that additional movement feels good (better than when you jump off your bed into those jeans that shrank in the dryer that you have to jump around or lie on your back and pray for good exhalation skills to zip).

You do not have to join a gym or participate in physical activity at a health club in order for it to "count." All physical activity during the day counts (except the finger and wrist movement of typing on a computer)! One of my best tips is to find five minutes every hour to get up and go for a walk. People look at me like I'm crazy, but people who still smoke always take their break to do something that we can all agree is unhealthy. Why not take your own break to get a short walk in? Why do we feel guilty doing something good for ourselves? So imagine that you work an eight-hour day. If you took a five-minute walk every hour, you would accumulate 40 minutes of physical activity during the day. Voilà! Just make sure you wear good footwear! If your athletic shoes are ten years old, it's time for a new pair. Likewise, flip-flops or stiletto heels aren't appropriate walking shoes.

Clearly, after seeking a doctor's approval, you can exercise. But let's face it—if you are ambulatory (which means you can walk on your own), you can start with something as basic as walking. During one of the shoots for *Honey We're Killing the Kids!,* I sat across the sofa from a morbidly obese dad who really didn't want to move. He wanted to know if he could walk the dog while driving the car! I told him that he should consider walking, that the physical activity would be good for him. He got very agitated and said to me, "My doctor didn't tell me to walk, he said to exercise. I can't exercise because I'm so fat." I explained that walking was a way to improve his ability to perform other exercise down the road. Often, physicians, while well intentioned, do not have enough information to provide to their patients to get them started on a physical fitness plan. I like to start with what you've got to work with and are willing to do!

RESOLVE TO EXERCISE

Is exercise regularly among your New Year's resolutions? If so, you're not alone. Ask any gym owner about their membership trends during the year. Gyms see the most people in January. Many people start the New Year off with good intentions that seem to fizzle out by the spring. However if you're determined to make this a lifestyle change, you need to:

- Think big, act small. Start with a vision of how you want to look and feel, but realize that you cannot transform yourself overnight. Take small steps to reach that goal. Exercise for 20 minutes, 3 times a week, and gradually increase to 30-40 minutes most days of the week.

- Set achievable goals. Set yourself up for success. If your schedule only allows three workouts a week, don't mentally commit to working out every day. Instead, aim for the three days a week, every week.

- Be **realistic.** Know your body's limits. Fitness is not an all-or-nothing endeavor. Don't give up if you get off track one day; just get back on course the next day.

SQUEEZING FITNESS INTO YOUR BUSY LIFESTYLE

Most busy people overestimate their physical activity level. They consider themselves active because they are always on the go. But while rushing from one meeting to another, or chauffeuring your kids to soccer practice, may make you feel like passing out from exhaustion, it's not the same as getting a sufficient amount of exercise.

You need a minimum of 60 minutes of physical activity every day. If you don't have a full hour to work out, remember that accumulation counts! Look for ways to capture opportunities to add more movement to your day. Cleaning the house, putting on music and dancing with the kids, doing yard work, and walking the dog are all good ways to boost your activity level. You'll soon notice that your energy and physical endurance will also increase.

There are also many ways to increase your muscle tone and

stamina without setting time aside for the gym. You can use your own body weight, or ordinary objects, as equipment. For example:

- Firm up those sagging, jiggling arms by doing arm curls while holding your pocketbook or groceries. Doing tricep extensions in the opposite direction uses opposing set of muscles.

- Use that same "equipment" to do arm raises by extending your arm out and bringing your hand up to shoulder height (no higher), and holding for five seconds at a time.

- Hold your infant while doing chest presses, shoulder raises and lunges.

- Instead of just sitting in that chair while watching TV, use it to do some squats. Picture yourself squatting over a dirty public toilet. You don't want to touch the seat. So you get down as low as possible, then stand up again. (Don't use your hands—keep them at your sides.)

- Do push-ups off a wall, counter or desk.

- A great leg exercise to do while sitting at your desk is to straighten your leg from a 90-degree angle while squeezing your quadriceps ("thighs"). Try to lift your leg a little higher before bringing it down.

- You can do abdominal exercises without lying on the floor. Sitting on the edge of the chair or sofa with your feet flat on the ground forces you to use your abdominal muscles to hold you up.

- Stuck in traffic or sitting in a meeting? Contract

("squeeze") your abdominal muscles and hold for a count of five before releasing.

- If the doctor is running late, take a fast-paced walk instead of sitting in the waiting room.

- Take the stairs instead of the elevator or escalator.

- In airports, walk–don't stand–on the moving sidewalks, or walk beside them.

- Use the park and playground equipment. Monkey bars are good for pull-ups. Pumping your legs while you swing is a great way to exercise your legs! To add even more resistance, try swinging with a toddler sitting on your lap and straddling your waist.

All of these little things can make such a big difference. Having better muscle tone and nicer posture enables you to carry yourself differently. If you are standing straighter with your shoulders back, your clothes will look better even if you haven't lost weight. It's like putting them on a hanger versus a hook.

I suggest you start by keeping a log of how many minutes each day you actually spend *moving*. Another option is to use a pedometer. It is a great way to measure steps. Soon your new activity level will become a habit, and you will realize that getting fit can be a realistic and attainable goal no matter how busy you are!

WORKOUT INTENSITY

You may have heard someone in passing talk about working out in their Target Heart Rate Zone. It is pretty simple to determine.

The general formula for the average person is:
220 – age x 60% (low)
220 – age x 90% (HRmax)
For example, a 30-year-old would calculate
her target zone using the above formula:
220 – 30 = 190. 190 x .60 = 114 and 190 x .90 = 171.
This individual would try to keep their heart rate
between 114 (low end) and 171 (high end) beats per minute.

The Karvonen Formula calculates your heart rate reserve range. To calculate it, take your pulse for one minute on three successive mornings upon waking up. Let's use a thirty-year-old female whose resting pulse was 69, 70 and 71, for an average of 70 over the three days.

Calculate her target heart rate by subtracting her age from 220 (220 – 30 = 190).

Subtract her average resting heart rate from her target heart rate (190 – 70 = 120).

The lower boundary of the percentage range is 50 percent of this plus your resting heart rate [(120 x .5) + 70 = 130]. The higher boundary is 85 percent plus your RHR [(120 x .85) + 70 =172]. Using the Karvonen Formula for percentage of heart rate reserve, this thirty-year-old woman should be working between 130 and 172 Beats Per Minute (BPM).

The above two formulas are only guidelines, as some people may be 30 beats above their predicted maximum heart rate. On the other end of the scale, some people can be 20 beats below, and will find it impossible to reach their so-called target zone. The best way, if you are interested, is to ask a qualified person who will monitor both you and your heart under exercise, and from this establish what your target zones should be.

Do you look at the numbers on the cardio equipment monitor? Another important factor is that results will vary by equipment and manufacturer, e.g., running and cycling. Don't worry if you don't have a Heart Rate Monitor. The Borg Scale of Perceived Exertion is another way of determining how hard you are working.

Using your own subjective Rate of Perceived Exertion (RPE) on a scale of 6–20 or a scale of 0–10, you determine how hard you "feel" you are working.

Original Scale	Revised Scale
6	0–Nothing at all
7–Very, very light	0.5–Very, very weak
8	1–Very weak
9–Very light	2–Weak
10	3–Moderate
11–Fairly light	4–Somewhat strong
12	5–Strong
13–Somewhat hard	6
14	7–Very strong
15–Hard	8
16	9–Very, very strong
17–Very hard	10–Maximal
18	–
19–Very, very hard	–
20–Maximal	–

The talk test is another good way of establishing how hard you are working. If you find it difficult to say a few words, you are probably working out anaerobically. For a good indication of aerobic exercise, you should be able to say a few words, catch your breath, and then carry on talking. If you are talking all the way through your workout without extra breaths, it's a good bet that you're not working hard enough.

TRAINING PANTS—BEGINNER EXERCISES FOR HOME

Lower Body
Quadriceps/Gluteals
Chair Squats
- Stand w/neutral posture and feet shoulder width apart & pointing forward
- Bend knees until buttocks touch seat
- Return to start position w/a smooth movement

Step-Ups
- Stand w/neutral spine, knees slightly bent, feet shoulder width apart
- Brace abdominals & step slowly up onto step
- Use the leg on step to lift body
- Lower body to start position using other leg

Hamstrings
Standing Leg Curl
- Stand w/neutral spine, feet shoulder width apart
- Hold onto chair w/hand

- Slowly curl leg toward buttocks
- Return to start position w/a smooth movement
- Repeat on opposite leg

Calves

Calf raises on step

- Stand w/balls of feet on step edge, knees slightly bent
- Support body w/hands on rail
- Raise heels to maximum height
- Slowly lower heels until a stretch is felt
- Maintain constant knee position

Upper Body

Chest

Push-ups on the wall

- Keep palms flat against wall, slightly wider than shoulder width apart
- Spine in neutral position
- Feet remain flat on the floor
- Slowly lean toward wall, bending at the elbows
- Pause, return to start position

Modified push-ups

- Support weight on hands & knees
- Keep trunk & thighs in line, spine in neutral position, abdominals braced
- Keep arms unlocked & hands slightly beyond shoulder width
- Bend arms to sides, lowering chest to just above floor level

- Push through arms, lifting chest until elbows are almost straight
- Ensure movements are smooth & controlled

Exercises with flexible resistance bands/dumbells

Chest

Chest Press (Resistance Band/Tubing)

- Wrap band behind back & wrap each end in each hand
- Bend elbows, hands in front of chest
- In controlled movement, push forward until elbows are completely extended
- Pause, then return to starting position

Back

Lat Pulldowns

- May be done with resistance band or dumbbells, in a seated or standing position
- Grip dumbbells or resistance band, palms forward, slightly wider than shoulder width above head
- Maintaining elbows out to sides, draw arms down in front of head to just above chest height
- Pause, return to start position

Seated Rows

- May be done with resistance-bands
- While sitting on the floor, wrap Resistance-Band around the bottom of your feet, gripping each end in each hand
- Hold at arms' length, elbows & knees slightly bent

- Keep trunk stabilized, spine in neutral & shoulders down
- Brace abdominals & pull toward lower chest, drawing elbows back & close to body
- Pause, extend arms back to starting position

Deltoids
Lateral shoulder raise
- Stand w/neutral posture, knees slightly bent
- Hold dumbbells at waist height, palms facing thighs
- Brace abdominals
- Raise arms slowly to horizontal
- Pause, then return smoothly to start position

Seated dumbbell shoulder press w/back rest
- Sit w/neutral spine, feet flat on floor & back supported
- Hold dumbbells at shoulder height, palms facing forward
- Brace abdominals
- Raise dumbbells vertically above shoulders
- Keep elbows slightly bent
- Slowly lower dumbbells to start position

Biceps
Dumbbell Biceps Curl
- Stand w/neutral posture, knees slightly bent
- Hold dumbbells, arms by sides, palms facing forward
- Keep shoulders still & bend elbows to raise dumbbells w/out moving trunk
- Return to start position slowly

Triceps

Triceps kick-backs

- Leaning on a flat surface with one leg up and bent, rest arm on knee
- Hold dumbbell, raise opposite elbow towards back
- Keep shoulder still & bend elbow to raise dumbbell without moving elbow
- Pause, then return smoothly to start position

Core

Abdominals

Crunches

- Lie on back, knees bent, feet flat
- Place fingertips behind ears, elbows out
- Curl upper body toward thighs slowly until trunk reaches a 45-degree angle
- Pause, lower shoulders slowly, uncurling spine
- Keep feet on floor as trunk goes down
- Do not bounce or "jerk" body

Abdominal bracing supine

- Lie on back, knees bent, feet flat
- Maintain neutral spine position
- Exhale slowly
- Draw lower abdominals toward spine
- Pause, then release muscle contraction

Half-curl down

- Sit on floor, spin in neutral, knees bent & heels drawn toward buttocks
- Extend arms out straight in front

- Allow pelvis to tilt backward, slowly lower trunk toward floor one vertebra at a time until 45-degree angle is reached
- Keep feet flat on floor
- Pause, return to starting position in a slow & controlled fashion, straighten spine while tilting pelvis forward

Quadruped abdominal bracing
- Begin in all-fours position, elbows slightly bent
- Maintain a neutral spine
- Exhale slowly
- Draw lower abdominals toward spine
- Maintain breathing using the diaphragm
- Pause, then release muscle contraction

Prone hold on elbows & knees
- Begin lying face-down propped on elbows, legs straight
- Maintain neutral spine position
- Brace abdominals
- Lift hips, support weight on elbows & knees
- Pause, then slowly return to start position

Spinal Erectors
Prone alternate arm & leg lift
- Begin lying face-down, arms at sides, palms facing down at shoulder level
- Maintain a neutral spine
- Lift one leg straight as high as possible, lifting the opposite arm (from the shoulders) as high

as possible, while keeping the rest of the
body down
- Pause, return to start position slowly

Bridging
- Lie on back, feet flat & arms by sides
- Brace abdominals to maintain neutral spine
- Slowly raise pelvis off floor to bring trunk & thighs in line
- Pause, return slowly to start position

Quadruped unilateral leg raise
- Begin on all fours position, elbows slightly bent
- Maintain neutral spine
- Exhale slowly
- Brace abdominals
- Slowly raise one leg to horizontal, maintain level hips, raise opposite arm
- Pause, then return to start position, release brace

Flexibility

Buttock
- Lie on your back w/knees bent
- Place one ankle on other knee
- Draw legs toward chest & grasp supporting knee w/ both hands
- Gently pull legs toward chest until you feel a stretch

Spinal Rotation
- Lie on back w/one leg straight
- Bring bent knee toward chest

- Grasp w/opposite hand
- Pull knee across toward floor
- Keep other arm out wide on floor w/shoulder down
- Look toward outstretched arm

Hip Bend
- Lie on back w/one leg straight
- Bend knee of other leg & gently pull it up toward chest
- Then pull knee toward opposite shoulder

Spinal Twist
- Sit on the floor
- Bend one knee & put the foot over the other thigh on floor
- Place opposite elbow on bent thigh, near knee
- Place other arm out behind to lean on
- Twist spine as push w/elbow
- Look over shoulder

Hamstring Sit
- Lean forward from hips
- Keep back & knee straight
- Reach toward toes

Hamstring Lying
- Lie on back w/knees bent
- Draw leg toward chest & straighten
- Gently bend foot toward you to stretch the sciatic nerve

- Hold stretch for a few seconds
- Release the toes & continue the muscle stretch
- Return to start position

Quads Stand
- Hold onto a chair
- Clasp foot w/opposite hand
- Draw knees backward

Quads Side Lie
- Clasp foot
- Pull thigh backward
- Keep knee in line w/hip

Front Hip
- Front foot well forward
- Hand on buttock of back leg
- Lean hips forward

Deep Calf
- Feet point forward
- Lower hips, bend knee
- Keep heel down
- Hold the stretch

Pecs + Wall
- Place forearm on wall or doorway
- Keep shoulder down
- Turn chest away from arm
- Be careful not to overstretch

Cat

- In all-fours position, tuck belly in & round back upward
- Push upward between the shoulder blades
- Tuck head & buttocks under toward each other
- Then relax & allow spine to hang downward
- Let chest & abdomen drop toward floor
- Lift head & buttocks upward

Roll-Up

- Lie on your back
- Bring knees toward chest
- Curl head & upper body
- Rock up & down rolling on spine
- Try to roll evenly & w/control

Slump Pull

- Round upper back, tuck in chest
- Place arm straight out in front
- Grasp wrist
- Pull arm forward & across
- Lean upper back backward

Triceps

- Place hand between shoulder blades
- Use other hand on elbow to pull it down & across
- Slide hand further down the back
- Hold the stretch for a few seconds
- Then lean upper body into the stretching side
- Push ribs out & upward

INTERMEDIATE/ADVANCED EXERCISES FOR HOME

Lower Body

Quadriceps/Gluteals

Dumbbell Squat

- Stand w/neutral posture, knees slightly bent & feet shoulder width apart & pointing forward
- Hold dumbbells by side & brace abdominals
- Bend knees until thighs are almost horizontal
- Keep feet flat on floor & maintain neutral spine position
- Return to start position w/a smooth movement

Static Lunge

- Stand in lunge position w/neutral spine, hands by side
- Brace abdominals
- Slowly lower hips toward floor
- Stop when front thigh is horizontal & front lower leg is vertical
- Return to start position w/a smooth movement

Dumbbell (Rear) Lunge

- Stand w/neutral posture, knees slightly bent, feet shoulder width apart
- Brace abdominals & slowly step backward
- Bend knees until front thigh is horizontal & front lower leg is vertical
- Return to start position w/a smooth movement

Dumbbell Step-Up
- Stand w/neutral spine, knees slightly bent, feet shoulder width apart & hold dumbbells by side
- Brace abdominals & step slowly up onto step
- Use the leg on step to lift body
- Return to start position by lower body using the leg on step

Core

Abdominals

Crunch—legs tucked
- Lie on back, feet off floor, knees bent toward chest, fingertips behind ears, elbows out
- Curl upper body toward knees slowly until trunk reaches a 45-degree angle
- Pause, lower shoulders slowly, uncurling spine as trunk goes down, keep legs still
- Do not bounce or "jerk" body

Bridging w/unilateral leg lift
- Lie on back, knees bent, feet flat and arms by sides
- Brace abdominals to maintain neutral spine
- Slowly raise pelvis off floor to bring trunk & thighs in line
- Raise one foot off floor, then straighten leg, keeping thighs parallel
- Pause, return slowly to start position

Crunches—legs vertical
- Lie on back, legs vertical, knees slightly bent, fingertips behind ears, elbows out

- Curl upper body toward thighs slowly until trunk reaches a 45-degree angle
- Pause, lower shoulders slowly, uncurling spine while maintaining leg position
- Do not bounce or "jerk" body

MANUAL RESISTANCE EXERCISES USING THERA-BAND OR RESISTANCE™ BAND

- **Flyes**—Hold resistance band out in front of you, bend arms slightly at the elbow and pull outward. **This exercise targets the chest.**
- **One-Arm Rows**—Tie resistance band to a doorknob, bend slightly at the waist, and pull arm back. Do one side at a time. **This targets the back.**
- **Reverse Flyes**—Hold resistance band in both hands and put band behind you this time. Bend arms slightly at the elbows and pull forward. **This targets the back.**
- **Side Lateral Raises**—Stand on resistance band, holding one end in each hand, bend knees slightly, and pull out to the sides. **This targets the top portion of the shoulders.**
- **Front Raises**—Same stance as above, but this time pull out in front of you. **This targets the front portion of your shoulders.**
- **Upright Rows**—Stand on resistance band, bend knees slightly, hold ends of band in each hand out in front of your waist. Keep wrists close together and pull up just under your chin. **This targets both front and side portions of your shoulders.**
- **Bicep Curls**—Stand on resistance band, one end in

each hand, knees slightly bent, pull both arms up simulating a bicep curl. **This targets the biceps.**

- **Kickbacks**–Tie one end of resistance band to a doorknob, hold other end in one hand, lean forward slightly, pull back and extend arm fully. **This targets the triceps.**

Advantages to using resistance bands are:
- they are relatively inexpensive in comparison with traditional weights
- they can be used anywhere, anytime (I keep one in my carry-on bag–you can easily put it in your pocketbook)
- the muscles can be worked maximally each repetition because of the constant resistance through the entire range of motion
- there is less of a chance of injury, since heavy weight is not being used

Here are the exercises that I used for the StairWELL Initiative during my doctoral research. We had pictures and instructions posted on the landing of each floor. You can get a pretty good total body workout from this regimen. However, if you add walking or jumping jacks for cardio, it would yield an even better result. Your body weight offers great resistance!

WALL SIT
- Place back to wall
- Legs should be hip width apart

- Slide down the wall slowly, until your knees are at a 90-degree angle—do not let your knees extend over your toes
- Slide up to the starting position

SHOULDER PRESS

Position A
- Stand with legs together
- Place tubing/band around stairwell pole slightly above your ankles' height
- Bend arms at your elbows—palms facing forward, arms along your sides, hands near your shoulders.

Position B
- Press up with your hands until your arms are straight
- Keep back straight
- Return hands to starting position

STANDING ROW

Position A
- Stand with legs shoulder width apart
- Place tubing/band around stairwell pole at your chest height
- Place arms directly in front of you

Position B
- Pull arms back, keeping elbows slightly below shoulder height

- Keep back straight (do not lean back)
- Return arms to starting position

BICEP CURL

Position A
- Stand with legs shoulder width apart
- Place tubing/band around stairwell pole slightly above your ankles' height
- Place arms directly in front of you, palms facing up

Position B
- Pull arms back, keeping elbows bent and at your sides (palms toward you)
- Keep back straight (do not lean back)
- Return arms to starting position

STEP DIP

Position A
- Sit on the step in order to create a 90-degree angle with your knees
- Hands are holding the edge of the step, knuckles facing forward (palms backward)

Position B
- Bring your body slightly forward and let your buttocks come down toward the lower step (do not sit on the step)
- Your elbows should bend behind you (not to the sides)
- Push up with your elbows to return to the starting position

LATERAL BRIDGE ON HAND

- Place hand on stair, supporting body at a 90-degree angle, opposite hand extended to the air
- Keep feet on the ground
- Hold for a count of 5 and then turn around and repeat with other arm

LATERAL BRIDGE ON HAND, ONE FOOT

- Place hand on stair, supporting body at a 90-degree angle, opposite hand extended to the air
- Raise one foot off the ground (feet hip width apart)
- Hold for a count of 5 and then turn around and repeat with other arm

WALL PUSH-UP

Position A

- Place arms firmly against wall, slightly wider than shoulder width
- Fingers should be pointing toward the ceiling
- Feet should be shoulder width apart

Position B

- Lean forward, keeping feet on the ground, back straight; Elbows should remain at shoulder height
- Push forward to return to starting position

STAIR PUSH-UP

Position A

- Place arms firmly on step, slightly wider than shoulder width

- Fingers should be pointing forward
- Feet should be shoulder width apart

Position B
- Lean forward, keeping feet on the ground, back straight; Elbows should remain at shoulder height
- Body should be parallel to the staircase
- Push forward to return to starting position

ABDOMINAL STABILIZER
Position A
- Sit on step with feet on the floor hip width apart
- Place hands on step with knuckles facing forward

Position B
- Lift right foot off the ground, hold for a count of 5
- Return foot to starting position

Position C
- Lift left foot off the ground, hold for a count of 5
- Return foot to starting position

Position D
- Lift both feet off the ground, hold for a count of 5
- Return feet to starting position

CALF STRETCH
Position A
- Place right foot against the step, toes up at a 45-degree angle, heel down
- Place hands on railing for light support/balance

Position B
- Come up onto left toe, leaning slightly forward
- Place hands on railing for light support/balance
- Repeat with opposite foot in front

QUADRICEPS STRETCH
- Place right hand on railing
- Bend left leg at the knee and grab the top of your foot with your left hand
- Keep back straight
- Hold for a count of 5 and repeat on opposite side

PIRIFORMIS STRETCH
Position A
- Sit on step
- Place right leg/foot over left knee
- Keep back straight

Position B
- Lean forward from the hip
- Do not round back
- Hold for a count of 5
- Repeat on opposite leg

HAMSTRING STRETCH
Position A
- Sit on step with left leg bent, right leg straight, foot flexed (toes pointing toward the ceiling)

Position B
- Extend right arm forward, left arm resting on left knee

- Attempt to touch right hand to right toes
- Hold for a count of 5 and repeat on opposite leg

LAT STRETCH

Position A

- Start with both hands wrapped around the bottom rail
- Keep feet hip width apart
- Bend forward from the hip, knees bent slightly

Position B

- Lean head forward
- Extend your buttocks back and bend forward at the waist
- Hold firmly to the rail for a count of 5

CHEST STRETCH

Position A

- Place right palm on the wall, fingers toward the ceiling
- Bend elbow and arm at 90-degree angle in line with the shoulder
- Keep feet hip width apart

Position B

- Rotate body away from the wall, leaning right shoulder forward
- Stretch (but not until it hurts) hold for a count of 5 and repeat on the opposite side

SHIN SPLINTS PREVENTION

Position A

- Sit on step with both knees bent at a 90-degree angle, hip width apart
- Keep feet flat on the floor
- Keep back straight

Position B

- Bend feet at the ankle
- Flex feet toward the ceiling
- Hold for a count of 5

SHIN STRETCH

Position A

- Hold on to the railing
- Right foot forward
- Bring left leg directly behind your body

Position B

- Bend both knees
- Do not extend right knee over the toes
- Place left sole of foot facing the ceiling
- Hold for a count of 5 and repeat on opposite side

REAR SHOULDER STRETCH

Position A

- Start with right hand extended directly in front of you, thumb pointed toward the ceiling
- Bend left hand and support right elbow

Position B
- Bring right arm across to the left side of your body
- Support right elbow with your left hand
- Hold for a count of 5 and repeat on opposite side

THIS JOKE'S FOR YOU!

Exercise is a great way to reduce stress. However, the easiest, most practical and affordable way to cope with stress is through LAUGHTER. It also can be aerobic in nature if you really get going. I know this because when I lived in New York City and went to comedy clubs, I laughed so hard that I needed my asthma inhaler!

Did you know????

- Females laugh more than males
- Children laugh 400 times a day, adults only 15
- 100 laughs = 10 minutes on a rowing machine
- 15 minutes of laughter = 8 hours of meditation
- 10 minutes of laughter = 2 hours of undisturbed sleep

More benefits of laughter:

- Boosts immune system
- Enhances creativity
- Increases circulation
- Decreases blood pressure
- Improves self-esteem
- Works facial, abdominal & respiratory muscles

Since we know laughter is great for your abdominal muscles,

I must recommend one last thing: use a stability ball in place of a chair while watching television, sitting at your desk or for exercise. It activates so many muscles in your body, especially your "core" to hold yourself up and remain stable! For sure you will laugh very hard if you keep falling off!

CHAPTER 8
Think Like a Skinny Person

Many years ago, I read an article that said that people who were thin were chronic dieters. I would have to agree with that to some extent. For the majority of people who are thin, life is about making choices: which jeans do you want to wear? If you consider that energy balance does not happen intuitively, then we as humans have to make choices, constantly, about what we eat and how much physical activity we will get in a day. Remember, we all have fat genes in our closet, so you can choose to make healthful choices most of the time and don't make the discretionary choices a daily occurrence. This will become a way of life for you. That is how you start to think like a skinny person and act like a skinny person—and before you know it, you are a skinny person!

For example, if we can agree that our eating should include consuming a significant amount of plant-based foods (fruits, vegetables and whole grains), then make sure you get them every day! Most of us are not getting our daily dose of fruits and veggies, and there is no pill or potion or superfood that can replace what we should be eating daily. Remember, these foods are not necessarily high in calories, but they do fill us up! Make a concerted effort to get your fruits in before dinner time. (They are fine to eat late. I'm just making a suggestion to get your fruit duty done earlier in the day so you don't forget it.) As for your veggies, start at lunch time (although I do love to rotate in some high-fiber V-8 juice in the morning) and make sure that by dinner you've consumed the minimum amount that you need.

One choice that I encourage my clients to make is to switch to skim milk and fat-free or low-fat dairy wherever possible. After the age of two, there is no reason why any of us need extra fat from dairy. I'm not saying you have to eat fat-free cheeses (heaven forbid—they taste like plastic), but by switching to skim milk and fat-free or low-fat yogurt you save the extra fat usually found in those dairy products for other foods in your day. (Don't put your hand between a piece of brie and my mouth or you will get bit!) This is why you can have pizza, ice cream and other typical diet no-no's with this plan. It's about moderation and choice. The same can be said for physical activity.

As with most behavior change, you need to set your goals. The key is to be realistic. For example, I would love to be 5'7", but it is unrealistic to think that other than a pair of three-inch heels, I will never obtain this height. I look at women in my yoga studio and secretly wish my thighs were thinner, but guess what? My genetic makeup will never permit me to look exactly like that. Better for me to focus on what I can control—my own yoga practice, which is making me stronger and healthier each day. So what is your reality? If you have 100 pounds to lose, can you do it? I certainly know you can! However, the key is to be realistic and set smaller sub-goals. In this case, look at your weight loss in 10-pound increments and celebrate each 10 pounds of weight loss with a non-food reward!

What are small changes you can make? Smaller portions, reducing calories, making better food choices (fiber is your friend), and increasing daily physical activity! This is the key to successful weight loss. If you wanted to run a marathon, would you just enter the race without training? I hope not, because 26.2 miles would not be fun if you didn't build up your endurance! In fact, it would be downright painful and even dangerous. This chapter will give examples of goal setting and modifying behaviors (like walking into the kitchen and sticking your head in the refrigerator when you get home) that can get in the way of our success. It will offer realistic strategies for successful change!

TIPS FOR LIVING WELL

Make a commitment to living in a healthful manner. We can each make improvements in our daily habits and behaviors that can have positive effects on our health and longevity. Instead of trying to change everything at once (and often failing to achieve all of your goals), set small, realistic, attainable goals. Once you've mastered one new achievement you can move on to your next goal. Here are some tips that I often recommend.

Eat closer to the earth.

This is another fancy way of saying—eat your fruits and vegetables! Most Americans do not get the *minimal* number of servings in each day (it's five). Try to incorporate fruit—fresh or dried—into you daily routine or as a snack between meals. As for veggies, we sometimes have to go out of our way to ensure that we eat any on a regular basis (let alone daily). There are so many varieties of fruits and vegetables that by exploring these food groups that come in a rainbow of colors, you are sure to keep meal time exciting! This also includes grains (which are plants).

Get up and move!

As humans, we were not meant to sit all day long. The heart is a muscle that needs to be worked every day! So, find ways to integrate more physical activity into your daily routine. As I said earlier, can you find a way to take a five-minute walk every hour? If you're at work for eight hours, that is 40 minutes of physical activity that you may not have been able to do at a gym at one point in time! We have all heard about taking the stairs vs. the elevator and choosing a parking spot further from our destination. Every little bit counts!

Drink more water!

The human body is 70 percent water, and water covers 71 percent of the earth! It is essential for normal body function—including transporting nutrients in the body, maintaining blood volume and regulating body temperature (to name just a few). Our society has increased its consumption of soft drinks and sodas over the last two decades—which often adds "empty" calories to our waistlines and can crowd out other foods that have nutritional value! The recommendations vary, but try to drink water instead of your other beverages!

Get a good night's sleep.

We forget that our bodies need to rest, renew and repair, and the best time to do this is when we are sleeping! Think of yourself like a recharging battery! We all function better after an evening of sound sleep! If you have difficulty sleeping, explore your evening rituals and try to ease into a gentle routine that will quiet your brain so you can slumber better.

I'm a big fan of daily multivitamin and mineral supplementation when you can remember to take it. This is a way to have a "security blanket" when it comes to your body's daily vitamin and mineral needs in case your food choices fall short! Remember, we have one body to get us through this thing we call life!

You should decrease caloric intake (although not too much) and increase your physical activity. Once again, making better food choices can help (eat more fruits, veggies and whole grains versus fried food and candy). Do not skip meals—that is one of the worst things you can do for your body. Instead, consider smaller portion sizes. Also, do not be fooled by calorie-free foods (including those with non-caloric sweeteners)—they may make you feel good temporarily, but they are not good for long-term health goals.

Finally, do not be driven by the numbers on the scale—there are other ways to measure your success: how do you feel in your clothes, what is your energy level, how is your skin, bowel habits, sleep habits, moods, etc.?

In my experience over the last decade, those who restrict

carbohydrates and rely on non-nutritive sweetners, are the people who crave sweets the most! Technically, all carbohydrates are "sugar." Do not demonize "sugar." Here's the scoop on sugar: it becomes glucose in your body, and glucose is your body's principal fuel source. We need it. Just don't let it be the only source of fuel. You need other nutrients too, and sugary foods often lack those. Look at those foods that are high in sugar and are just not very nutritious—check the labels of candy, soft drinks, cakes, pies, ice cream, etc., and see for yourself. Once in a while it's okay to have these super sugary foods—but not daily. And of course, sugar also promotes tooth decay.

If you like sweet-tasting foods (and most of us do), I encourage you to make nutrient-rich, high-fiber choices such as fruits, vegetables, and whole grains. Your healthy diet can also include occasional less-healthy foods as well, but make them special treats after you've met your caloric and nutritional needs.

Keep in mind that sugar is extremely prevalent in our food supply, and goes by many names, including sucrose, fruit juice, high fructose corn syrup, honey, brown sugar, molasses, lactose (in dairy) and more. At the end of the day, it's all sugar.

YOU CAN EAT AFTER 7 P.M.

Avoiding food in the evening hours is a good strategy if you go to bed at 8:00 p.m., but try to remember the last time you did that! The point is, your body doesn't stop functioning according to the time of the day. Your organs and tissues are working hard around the clock, and they rely on fuel. If you last eat at 6 p.m. and don't eat again until 8 a.m., that is a 14-hour fast. You wouldn't do that during the day, would you? Don't forget that the brain is an organ, too, and relies on fuel just as your muscles do.

For those who, like myself, tend to be up late at night, eating in the evening is the only way to keep my brain and other organs primed for work. All calories do not magically get deposited in your "fat" saddlebags while you sleep. In fact, you burn more fat for fuel during rest—and sleep is the ultimate form of rest. A good night's sleep is critical to allow your body to rest, repair, and renew itself.

You should, though, try not to eat and lie down immediately afterward, which can cause reflux of digestive acids into the esophagus—a.k.a heartburn—and interfere with restful sleep.

DO SNACK BETWEEN MEALS

Eating every two to three hours—five or six times per day—has three important benefits. First, it helps maintain your blood sugar levels, especially if each feeding includes adequate carbohydrates. Moderate dips in blood sugar levels can make you tired, irritable and listless. Second, frequent feedings keep you from overeating at mealtimes. Your brain, mouth, and stomach have a communication breakdown when you're ravenous. As a result, you inhale too many calories before you realize that you've met your hunger needs. Finally, the act of eating burns calories, so by consuming food at more frequent intervals you keep your metabolism revved up all day long. For this reason you should never skip meals; you'll only slow down your metabolism.

Don't make the mistake, though, of mindlessly noshing all day long, which can lead to overeating and poor food choices. Instead, plan your snacks just as you do your meals. Savor your food, chewing slowly so that your brain has time to receive the message that you are full.

DON'T WORRY ABOUT FOOD COMBINATIONS

These days, bookstore shelves are lined with fad-diet books touting complex eating formulas. The foundation of many of these regimens is a prohibition against mixing various foods and food groups—carbs and proteins, simple carbs and complex ones, fruits and vegetables, and so on. The human body is a pretty awesome machine, and it knows how to handle just about any combination of foods you feed it.

WATERPROOF JEANS?

How much water do you need to drink? The research changes every year, but the simple recommendation to replace what is lost is the best. Fluids leave our bodies during respiration, perspiration, urination and defication. You still need to drink water because it is essential to life and comprises 70 percent of the human body. You know you're well hydrated if your urine is plentiful, pale or clear in color. If it's scant or dark yellow, you need to drink more fluids.

Consuming beverages with non-caloric sweeteners only seems to perpetuate our behavior and drive toward sweets. We can and should modify our intake. When you consume fluids, they should have some value—water, milk, 100 percent fruit juice, tea, coffee or club soda.

DON'T BUY INTO THE "LONGEVITY DIET"

You may have heard recently that cutting calories can help you live longer. The problem with that claim is that the research that supports it was conducted on lab animals. When the critters were fed diets that contained only 60 percent of their normal caloric intake, they lived 50 percent longer. Human volunteers are currently participating in research conducted at the National Institute on Aging, but it will be years before results are known. In the animal studies, the subjects that consumed less food experienced less oxidative stress in the brain, which theoretically would decrease their risk for Alzheimer's, Parkinson's, and Huntington's diseases, and stroke. This may be a health-promoting mechanism in humans as well.

However, research by Jing Fang, MD, at the Albert Einstein College of Medicine at Yeshiva University, found increased rates of deaths from heart disease in people who consumed diets as low as 1,100 calories per day. These results suggest that eating more and exercising to maintain a healthy weight may actually help you to live longer. Remember what I suggested earlier; eat at least 1,200 calories per day!

What about periodic fasting, something also being touted in the media? Some research has found fasting to be more effective than exercise at lowering heart rate and blood pressure. However, the benefits of healthy eating and regular exercising have long been documented as being the most effective strategies for health promotion. Throughout history, some people have fasted for spiritual reasons, and that is their choice and prerogative. One practice I definitely do not recommend is fasting to flush toxins from the body or to try and lose a few pounds quickly.

The best strategy is to eat when you are hungry and stop when you are full.

DON'T LOOK FOR A MAGIC PILL

If there really were a pill to increase muscle mass, speed up metabolism, burn excess calories, or improve athletic performance, we'd all be taking it and the manufacturers would be billionaires. To feel and look your best, you need to eat well and exercise regularly—it's as simple as that. There is no shortcut.

Have you ever thought that because a weight-loss product or herb is natural that it is safe and effective? Well, my favorite "natural" plant to mention in this category is arsenic. It does not help you to lose weight. It is a plant, it is "natural," and it is also a poison that can kill you. So, it's not safe! In 1994, the Dietary Supplement and Health and Education Act (DSHEA) made it the "wild west" with selling non-prescription products with "natural" claims by limiting the FDA's ability to regulate these products. Just because it says that it is safe doesn't mean that it is. I had an acquaintance from the gym who died after taking an over-the-counter product that contained Ephedra. He lost over 40 pounds in less than four months, and then went to take a nap after a workout and never woke up. Is it really worth it? How many people have consumed diet teas and died? Was it really worth it? Even if it's a prescription, it doesn't mean its safe. Look at the fate of Fen-phen. It was finally pulled after people died and many more went on to have chronic heart problems. There are people who, to this day, are very upset that they can no longer get this drug combination for weight loss. Is it worth your life or health? You have one body, and as far as we know, one lifetime to use it. Remember, safe, effective and sustained weight loss is not about shortcuts and quick fixes. What has been tried and true really is the secret to success and arguably longevity. You can't get that stone-washed look over night!

Truth be told, "Skinny" girls make different food choices! Here are some suggestions for healthy trade-offs. That simple spoonful of mayonnaise or little pat of butter on your snack isn't as innocent as it seems. Try substituting some healthier trade-offs instead of your usual choices!

In place of...	Substitute	Calories saved	Fat grams saved
2 oz potato chips	2 oz pretzels	74	18
1 c. whole milk	1 c. skim milk	50	7
2 choc. chip cookies	2 ginger snaps	44	4
1 croissant	1 bagel	85	11
1 slice carrot cake	1 slice angel food cake	260	21
1 c. sour cream	1 c. yogurt	355	41
1 all-beef frankfurter	1 chicken frankfurter	45	5
1 bacon cheeseburger	1 plain hamburger	219	16
3 oz French fries	1 medium baked potato	54	14
1 oz chocolate	1 oz gumdrops	45	9
1 tbs. mayonnaise	1 tbs. mustard	85	10
2 oz American cheese	2 oz mozzarella	50	8
2 c. popcorn cooked in oil	2 c. air-popped popcorn	50	5
1 tbs. butter	1 tbs. fruit preserves	45	12
3 oz roast beef	3 oz roast turkey	225	30

Here are some tips to get you through the winter holidays—
and remember: there are 11 more months to go!

- Don't go to a party hungry—hunger leads to overeating. Drink some juice, eat a piece of fruit, have a handful of almonds or some crackers before leaving.
- Don't stand around the food table; take the foods you want and leave the area.
- Watch alcohol intake—alcohol drops your resistance and can result in overeating. Drink a glass of water between alcoholic beverages. Skip beer. Drink vodka, tequila, gin, or wine to get the maximum buzz for your calorie budget.
- If the party calls for you to bring something, make it a low-cal item. That way you know you can load up on it.
- Engage people in conversation—it's hard to talk and eat at the same time. Talking slows your eating and helps you recognize when you're full.
- Don't skip once-a-year favorites—skipping them can lead to frustration and deprivation. Instead, enjoy smaller portions.
- Decide which foods hold special meaning for you, which foods you love the most, and which foods you can live without. Once you have decided, skip the least favorite and focus on smaller portions of the higher-calorie favorites.
- Increase your physical activity. After your meal, have the family take a walk together.

LEARN HOW TO USE FOOD SUBSTITUTIONS FOR HOLIDAY DINNERS

- Use evaporated skim milk in place of cream. You can whip it and use it in sauces, casseroles and even the pumpkin pie.
- Applesauce fills in for oils in baked goods. Try equal amounts of it in muffins, breads, cakes and cookies.
- Fruit juice is a good base for salad dressing or marinade.
- Cocoa powder works in brownies, cakes and fudge; just use three tablespoons for every ounce of unsweetened chocolate.
- Use Greek (strained) Fat-free yogurt in place of sour cream for dips, recipes and potatoes!
- Try hummus in the place of mayonnaise to lubricate a sandwich or hold tuna, chicken or turkey salad together!

Start with dips—use fat-free sour cream or fat-free yogurt for the base. Yogurts increase nutrition while decreasing fat. For dippers, try veggie sticks and baked pita squares. Fat-free sour cream or yogurt can be used in salad dressings. There are lots of options to think about once the main course is out of the way. For turkey stuffing, moisten bread crumbs with fat-free broth; bake the stuffing outside of the bird to keep calories down and keep the stuffing safe from bacteria. Always strain the fat from chicken soup! Include lots of vegetables, both cooked and raw, and fresh or dried fruit. Steam vegetables, then season with herbs, nuts, herbs, lemon or a small amount of parmesan cheese for flavor. Buy both white and sweet potatoes to provide flavor variety and a low-fat option. Remember, potatoes are not inherently fattening—it's what you put on them that can cause you to exceed your calorie budget.

Green leaf or romaine lettuce for the salad and a mix of chopped fresh vegetables can help to keep nutritional balance. Try an apple salad, stewed apples, or even orange segments mixed with greens to increase fiber as a low-fat choice. Toss sunflower seeds on your salad to add protein. Don't forget cranberries—they are great in salads, grain or rice dishes, hot cereal, and turkey sandwiches!

As for dessert, make pies without the crust. Pumpkin, pecan, apple and blueberry fillings have all the flavor anyway. If you need whipped cream, try a low-fat or fat-free version.

Aunt Marilyn's Apple Crisp

6 sliced/peeled/cored Granny Smith apples.

¾ cup brown sugar

¾ cup whole wheat flour

½ cup butter

1. In an 8-ounce square glass baking dish, combine the apples; cut into small pieces (not pureed).
2. On top of the sliced apples, place a mixture of the brown sugar, whole wheat flour, and butter (the mixture will be crumbly).
3. Bake at 350° until the apples are soft and the top is brown (about 30–45 minutes).
3. Serve warm (add a dollop of vanilla Greek yogurt instead of ice cream on top).

QUICK-TO-FIX MEAL TIPS

"Live Skinny" and prepare your own food. When time is short, don't give up on the healthful eating. Just take some shortcuts to save time and energy.

Plan ahead

Prepare ingredients ahead of time. For example, wash and trim broccoli florets. Skewer kebabs with veggies and meat pieces the night before. Cook lean ground meat ahead for soft tacos.

Stock your pantry with quick-to-fix foods

Include pasta, rice, frozen and canned veggies, canned fruits, bread, lean deli meats, salad ingredients, salsa, canned beans, milk, yogurt, and cheese.

Buy prepared foods

For example, try grated cheese, pre-cut stir-fry veggies, shredded cabbage, skinless chicken strips, mixed salad greens, prewashed spinach and chopped onion. Even thin-sliced, lean deli meat is quick for stir-fried recipes or slapping together a sandwich.

Keep a variety of prepared foods on hand

Check the Nutrition Facts panel on the food label to choose those that match your nutrition needs. Prepare them along with fresh foods: for example, prepared pasta sauce heated with cooked ground meat, then served over pasta or a microwave-baked potato.

When you have time to cook, make a double or triple batch

For example, simmer enough pasta for two days. Divide it

into two parts: serve it hot one night w/meat sauce, then the remainder chilled as a salad w/tuna, dill & low-fat salad dressing the next day.

Cook on weekends

Save food "prep" time on weekdays. Freeze leftovers in individual containers for quick thawing mid-week.

Use quick-cooking methods

Stir-frying, broiling and microwaving are usually faster than baking or roasting. Slice meat and poultry in thinner slices for faster cooking.

Prepare meals that pack variety in just one dish

Try chicken fajitas in a soft taco. Stuff tuna and vegetable salad into a pita pocket. Prepare a ham and spinach quiche. Make a chef's salad, which requires no cooking at all.

Serve assemble-your-own menus

These include deli sandwiches, mini-pizzas on English muffins, or burgers with veggies and cheese toppings.

CHAPTER 9
Preventing Your Genes from Getting Stained (Society/Those Who Sabotage Efforts)

● ●

When we look good in our jeans, somebody is apt to be jealous—or at least envious! It is bad enough that there are things around us that sabotage our efforts: fast food, fat food, promises of miraculous weight loss in pills and potions, sedentary jobs, long and exhausting days of being über-people—even well-meaning parents, employees, friends, and siblings. Some research suggests that if we surround ourselves with fat friends, we will become fat! Our friends can make us fat? I think that is nonsense—there are fat people everywhere! For anyone who thinks that between work and their lives they cannot "win" this battle, I say: bring it on.

First, you need to let the people around you know that you need their help. Let's face it: if you had cancer and required assistance with your treatment, everyone around you would be sympathetic and help you. If you had a serious food allergy that would cause you to go into anaphylactic shock, most people who know you well would NOT serve it to you (at least I hope not)! What is my point? Ask people around you—family members, friends and co-workers—to help you.

I had one client tell me that her brother would bake pies and cakes to taunt her, until she finally said, "Listen—you know I've been struggling with my weight, to the extent that I have trouble even leaving my house. Please help me instead of hurting me." He then became her hiking and walking buddy and didn't bake quite as often. During my doctoral research, we had departments at the university stop putting candy out in the office and replace it with dry-roasted, unsalted almonds. How many times have you ever bought the candy on sale, after a holiday (because it was a deal) and brought it to your home or office to nosh on? It just is not necessary, and we sabotage the efforts of those around us by leaving those foodstuffs out.

I live in a family of people with fat genes. As an adult, I have chosen to prepare many holiday meals, which have been rich in tradition but not in calories or fat. I always offer loads of healthier foods and there is always dessert in my house, just not overwhelming quantities of it.

STAYCATION, ANYONE?

During tough economic times, people spend less on travel, just as they may have cut back on buying new threads. I have suggested that we take lessons from the reality-show world when it comes to weight loss—who can make working out a full-time job when you have a full time job? It may be challenging to find the time and the resources to be good to yourself in order to help you achieve your health goals. So consider this option: take the money you would spend on a vacation (in most cases, this is still less expensive), and make the week (or two) all about you! Clear out your pantry and buy healthy foods. If you don't know how to cook—take a cooking class or have a personal chef come to your home to teach you. Consider hiring a personal trainer for a week of training sessions. Plan daily physical activity that can be spread out throughout the day—a vigorous workout, then add on walking, biking, swimming, hiking—depending on the season and resources in your community. And for an extra treat, just like at a spa, add yoga, meditation, a manicure, pedicure, haircut, or massage.

Activities & Rewards to Substitute for Eating

Instead of using food as a reward for a hard day's work or because you're upset, do other things for yourself.

- Attending sporting events
- Enjoying leisure activities
- Exercising or playing sports
- Gardening
- Getting praise from others

- Going to a movie or play
- Listening to music
- Manicure/pedicure
- Massage
- Napping
- Praising yourself
- Reading
- Receiving token rewards
- Redecorating
- Relaxing
- Saving money for future treats
- Shopping
- Spa visit
- Taking a bubble bath
- Telephoning friends and family
- Tidying your room or house
- Vacationing
- Working on hobbies or crafts

SURVIVING THE WINTER HOLIDAY SEASON

Every year, there are articles on this very subject: how to enjoy all the food-centered holidays without putting on too much weight and throwing away all sense of reason when it comes to nutrition and your health goals. It seems that this season starts at Halloween and continues through Valentine's Day! Maybe subconsciously we are getting ready to hibernate for the winter. It is difficult to lose weight during this time of year. So it is better to aim for weight maintenance if you find your weekends are filled with parties.

My first recommendation: do not think of going on a diet

this time of the year. Instead think of that "d" word as "**Did I Eat That?**" Here are some ways to ensure you do not over eat during the holidays:

- Do not starve yourself all day long—this will set you up to binge when you show up at the party; you will overeat whatever is in front of you.
- Plate all your food, which means put everything you are going to eat on one plate (even when there are appetizers/nosh) and only eat what is on that plate; this way you can keep track of your portions.
- Have a little taste of everything—a fork or spoonful (even dessert).
- When sitting down to your meal, make sure half your plate has vegetables on it, one quarter of your plate has a starch/grain and the last quarter of your plate has your protein (chicken, turkey, beef, fish, etc.).
- Put your fork down between bites—this will help to slow you down, so your stomach will not become overfilled before your brain gets the message to stop.
- Beware of the calories you drink, both in alcohol and other season beverages; alternate with water or club soda.
- When cooking, try to use less fat/oil than the recipe calls for.
- Pace yourself. I learned that the hard way. The first time my aunt's mother had me over for the traditional Italian, seven-fish Christmas Eve dinner, I thought I was going to explode!

- Don't forget to move around and keep physical activity part of your everyday routine!
- Do not buy bags of holiday candy—it sabotages everyone's efforts to combat the battle of the bulge. Instead, put out dried fruit and nuts!

I absolutely love to host the holidays at my home. For me, cooking is about sharing my passion for food, providing nourishment to my friends and family, and my way of bestowing love on the people in my life! I strive to prepare foods that are nutritious and flavorful. My secret is to prepare a lot of side dishes, which are, of course, mostly vegetables and whole grains!

ADD DRIED FRUIT

Raisins, cranberries, blueberries and cherries can be a wonderful addition to any dish—from a salad to a grain dish. Dried fruit really packs big flavor, antioxidants, fiber, vitamins and minerals when added to your dish! You can add dried fruit to your family's stuffing recipe.

I am known for my famous "turkey"—whether it's just the breast or the whole thing. My secret seasoning is Chef Paul Prudhomme's Poultry Magic. Pat it on the turkey (or chicken)—no need for oil or butter. Fill the pan with apple cider, pearl onions, pitted dates, figs, and chestnuts. Baste as needed. After the turkey is done, take the fluids and solids out of the pan; use a separator to remove the oil/fat. Use a hand blender to puree, and voilà—you have a thick gravy made from wholesome ingredients that tastes great!

SNEAK IN FAT-FREE YOGURT

Many of us like to dip chips, veggies and even our food into something! I frequently use the Greek style fat-free yogurt for a variety of dips. A Lebanese friend taught me how to make labneh—which simply includes using strained yogurt, a few drops of olive oil and some sea salt. Really easy to make. Now, to enhance that, I add Z'atar seasoning (after once finding it prepared that way). You can always use fat-free yogurt for just about any recipe that calls for sour cream. Add your own blend of seasoning to it! When I make a salmon dish, I usually prepare lemon cups and place on each plate as follows:

Halve lemons and drain the juice. Remove the pulp and cut a small piece from the bottom of each half (skin side) in order for the lemon half to "sit" on the plate without rolling.

Combine lemon juice, fresh dill and Greek yogurt in a bowl. Then fill each lemon "cup" with the mixture.

Your guests will think they are eating something that is rich in calories—but you know it's simply rich in flavor and nutrients! Lemons are loaded with vitamin C, iron, calcium, magnesium, phosphorous, potassium and zinc.

FORGET THE FADs (FAST ACTING DIETS)

What is a fad diet? A fad is defined by www.dictionary.com as "A fashion that is taken up with great enthusiasm for a brief period of time; a craze." The same website defines diet as "The usual food and drink of a person or animal" and adds, "A regulated selection of foods, as for medical reasons or cosmetic weight loss." So we could say that a fad diet is the food and drink of a person taken up with great enthusiasm for a brief period of time. Well, I prefer to suggest that regardless of your health goals, the eating habits that you develop now should be adequate to take you through the remainder of your life.

In springtime, people start to become more aware that swimsuit season is rapidly approaching. In an effort to look one's best in less time, many attempt to use fad diets as a quick-fix solution. However, most individuals see some fast results that usually cannot be maintained for any length of time. It is true that each person's body is unique, but what our bodies need for fuel, function, repair and renewal is the same: we need carbohydrates, protein, fat, water, vitamins, minerals and fiber for overall health and well being.

Okay, so what should you eat? Get back to basics: eat "whole" foods, which basically means foods that closely resemble the way they are found in nature. Fruits, vegetables, low-fat dairy, lean protein, fats (from plants and animals vs. the fried variety), and grains. For more information on healthy eating guidelines, go to www.MyPyramid.gov, where you can find out your unique caloric intake needs and what that means in food servings. You will also find information about physical activity (which is the other half of the equation).

So where does the weight loss come in? Well, it's real simple—the answer is balance. Changes in weight are related to energy expended versus energy consumed. So if you are trying to lose weight, you need to eat fewer calories than you burn. The opposite is true for gaining weight. While some programs and plans make promises of speedy weight loss, it generally is accounted for by loss of "water weight." It looks great on the scale, but is not a true loss of body fat (which is what we're really looking for). The best way to get rid of the fat is to exercise—not just for burning calories, but to work on toning up muscles (you look leaner even if the numbers on the scale aren't going down as rapidly). Remember, the only person who sees the numbers on the scale is YOU. I often tell my patients not to worry about the numbers and to measure success in other ways—how do your clothes feel, how is your energy level, do you feel full?

Finally, your overall health and well-being are important for feeling good over time. So remember, eating nutrient-rich foods can be an important part of decreasing your risk factors for heart disease and some cancers.

How do you identify a fad diet? We have discussed some ways to narrow in on a fad, but here are some more:

- Suggests taking supplements, shakes, vitamins, minerals or herbal remedies to account for losses in the diet.
- Assigns labels to foods such as "good" or "bad."
- Uses "testimonials" by individuals and/or celebrities.
- Attempts to discredit dietetics professionals.
- Claims to cure ailments and/or provide "spot" reduction of body fat in certain body compartments.
- Blames hormones for weight problems.
- Eliminates a food group.

While there is not one diet or eating plan that works best for all people, I would suggest that you make your food choices based upon the recommendations of the U.S. Department of Agriculture (USDA) and the National Institutes of Health

(NIH). While many of the authors and/or creators of these books, plans and programs try to discredit the nutrition information provided by these well-respected organizations, their principles are based upon science and do not benefit from the sales of books, supplements, shakes, videos, or other products. My recommendations for meal planning integrate the principles because they have been proven over time to be safe and effective!

You will have a first-rate eating plan if you eat a diet that is made up of:

- Foods from each of the food groups
- Adequate servings of fruits and vegetables (at least 5 servings combined each day)
- At least 3 servings per day of low-fat or fat-free dairy products
- Whole grains and low-fat protein
- At least 8 glasses of water each day

FUN WITH SUMMER PRODUCE

Living in the Garden State, I have access to amazing produce that is grown right in our own backyards (literally)! When the weather is warm, we are often more open to eating healthier—especially since we can barbeque and eat outdoors. In addition to enjoying what is fresh and in season at the moment, I often encourage my clients to buy produce in bulk when the prices drop.

Fruits and vegetables not only add flavor to your meals, they also create a rainbow of colors which make mealtime visually as well as gastronomically pleasing. Research shows that people who eat more fruits and vegetables have a decreased risk for certain cancers (like colon cancer). For people who are watching their weight, fruits and vegetables are a great way to pack in nutrient-dense foods, which are also lower in calories (assuming you are not drowning them with fat)! Summer fruits, and some vegetables, have lots of water, which is what we need more of during the hot months to keep our bodies well-hydrated! Produce also contains fiber, which fills you up, helps to lower cholesterol, and helps to keep your gastrointestinal tract in shape!

A fun way to cook your veggies is to marinate them and throw them on the barbeque grill! Another easy way to cook is to wrap your veggies and meat/poultry/fish in aluminum foil pouches, which keeps the flavors "locked" together while preventing charring. This can be done in an oven or barbeque.

Blueberries

Loaded with antioxidants, this versatile summer fruit can be thrown in salads, yogurt, cereal, pancakes, muffins, cookies, on top of ice cream, pies, over angel food cake—you get the idea. Blueberries contain vitamin B6, vitamin C, vitamin K and fiber! Blueberries have antioxidants in the pigments—referred to as phytochemicals—which may have anti-cancer and heart-healthy properties like polyphenols and resveratrol. Here is a breakfast parfait:

4 oz Greek-style vanilla yogurt (0% fat)
1/3 cup Kellogg's All-Bran Bran Buds
1/2 cup of fresh blueberries

When the price of blueberries drops, load up on them by the pint. Wash and freeze them in small bags to use throughout the year. Great in pancakes (made with whole grains or Fiber One Bran Cereal) or smoothies.

Tomatoes

I won't lie—I'm a Jersey Girl, and I'm partial to our tomatoes, but many people enjoy growing tomatoes on their own. Technically, tomatoes are a fruit, even though they aren't sweet like berries! Tomatoes are best known for lycopene; they also contain vitamins A and C. I am a particular fan of the heirloom varieties in the summer because of the different colors and flavors. Tomatoes are such a versatile food—used in salads, stews, gravy, omelets, soups, salsa, on sandwiches or alone. I always purchase large quantities of tomatoes and make tomato sauce and freeze it (or can it). One fun way to make marinara is to make "sunshine sauce": use all yellow: tomatoes, peppers, onions; add garlic and parsley, oregano, basil, salt and white pepper. You can use ground flax seed in lieu of tomato paste to thicken the sauce! This is great over warm pasta or even mozzarella!

Here is a recipe for a wonderful spread to complement fresh tomatoes:

In a food processor combine: 1 cup tightly packed basil, 1/2 cup fat-free ricotta, 6 oz of feta cheese (low-fat or fat-free if available). Chop, then pour in olive oil until it has the consistency of yogurt. Add a dollop to sliced tomatoes.

This bruschetta recipe is great as a salsa-type dip, on bread/crostini, served chilled atop grilled chicken or fish (like swordfish). You can use any tomatoes that suit your fancy. Chop them up, add some fresh diced garlic, fresh chopped basil, olive oil, salt and pepper to taste.

Corn

We all know that nothing tastes as good as local corn in August and September. I actually buy it by the bushel when it's in season and freeze it. My grandmother taught me how to truly appreciate the flavors of foods. As I was about to rub an ear of corn with butter and salt, my Grandma Jeannette stopped me and said, "Felicia, do you have any idea what that corn really tastes like? It has flavor that is really unique. Eat it plain so that it doesn't just taste like butter and salt." From that moment on, I learned to appreciate the sweet flavor of fresh corn. I am willing to forgo eating it when it's not in season, because once you've had the best, you don't want the rest.

While many people think of corn as a starch, it is a really a vegetable! It also has a lot of insoluble fiber so, as I tell my clients, you burn a lot of calories moving the corn from your mouth through your digestive tract and out of your body! Corn contains vitamin C, and one medium ear of corn has about 75 calories. It also is loaded with lutein, and also zeaxanthin, an antioxidant cousin to beta-carotene (vitamin A).

One of my favorite ways to make corn on the cob is simply to steam it with water and splash of skim milk. Cook on high heat for 7 to 8 minutes. The lactose in the milk enhances the sweet taste. I always make enough for dinner and then some extra to eat cold the next day. (We can be seen at the beach with ears of cold corn in our hands!)

Melons

Whether it be watermelon, honeydew or cantaloupe—melons are truly nature's candy! These summer fruits are packed with flavor and water! You can create a rainbow fruit salad using different-colored melons (and adding those summer berries)!

The way I keep melons ready to eat for my family is to take a melon baller and scoop the moist flesh out of the melon and keep it in a container. How often do we look at the melon and are not in the mood to cut it up? This is a great way to make melon a grab 'n go fruit! You can also put the melon balls in the freezer and use them in a smoothie (or to chill a summer cocktail). Melons can also be nice for making fruited waters for yourself and guests.

Some people enjoy melon and prosciutto. You can also use melon when you kebab veggies and meat, poultry or fish on the grill.

Melon Salsa

1½ cups of diced melon

½ cup of diced pineapple

¼ cup of finely diced red onion

2 tablespoons of minced fresh cilantro

2 tablespoons of olive oil

1 tablespoon of raspberry vinegar

1 tablespoon of lemon juice

¼ teaspoon of cayenne pepper

½ teaspoon of finely minced garlic

½ teaspoon of honey

Salt and black pepper, to taste

Combine the diced melon, diced pineapple and red onion. In another bowl, whisk together the olive oil, vinegar, lemon juice, cayenne pepper, garlic and honey; then season with salt and pepper. Before serving, combine the two mixtures and gently toss with the cilantro.

Enjoy the rich flavors of the summer and know that you are treating your body to a rainbow of vitamins, minerals and phytonutrients! Who says foods that taste good aren't good for you?

WHAT TO DO WHEN YOU'RE AT THE MALL

When it's getting chilly outside and you have time to do some holiday shopping, or you're escaping the heat of the summer, what should you eat when at the mall? The question is, "What are the best food choices to make when dining out?"

There are many really great options for food at your local shopping mall. In addition to the traditional fast-food restaurants, there are some chains that can be found only at large shopping centers. Remember, just as holiday eating can be a challenge, dining out with your friends does not have to be a contest of overconsumption. Even when you are dining out, consider the types of foods you have or have not consumed for the day. For example, if it's dinner time and you haven't had any vegetables yet, you might consider veggies on your pizza or a large salad with grilled chicken. And don't forget, many fast-food chains now sell fruit.

I would never tell you that you can never have fast food—but remember, you do not need to supersize or get the largest portions that are available. Consider ordering your sandwich with the small fries (or salad) and, in lieu of soda, bottled water. Salads are a great choice when they are not swimming in dressing. Remember, you can hold the mayonnaise and use barbeque sauce, ketchup or mustard for flavor!

Better Fast-Food Options

- Single slice of veggie pizza
- Grilled, not fried, sandwich (for example, a grilled chicken breast sandwich) or salad
- Small hamburger or cheeseburger
- Rotisserie chicken
- Deli turkey sandwich
- Bean burrito
- Baked potato
- Chili (go easy on the cheese & skip the sour cream)
- Small French fries
- Bottled water
- Salad, side or regular, but watch the dressing, chips and croutons!
- Frozen yogurt
- Reduced-fat ice cream
- Fruit salads

There are always several ethnic cuisines represented at the food court that offer healthy options. Just remember that portion size counts—and avoid the fried stuff!

Italian

- Small order of pasta with marinara
- Meatballs
- Salads (go easy on the dressing)

Greek

- Greek salad
- Gyro
- Falafel

Japanese

- Sushi
- Miso soup
- Edamame

Chinese

- Brown rice
- Mixed vegetables
- Soup (wonton, egg drop, hot 'n sour)

Everything in moderation is fine. Remember, it's just food. Food is meant to be pleasurable and enjoyed—but a Saturday night at your local mall will not be your last supper! One of my favorite aspects of going to the mall is the great distance that you can potentially walk and take the stairs (instead of elevators and escalators). For kicks, try a pedometer to see how many steps you take when you're cruising around!

Just because you're cutting down on fat and salt doesn't mean your taste buds have to take a vacation from flavor. A creative cook can make low-fat, low-sodium cooking exciting, imaginative and crowd-pleasing. Here are a few great flavor-enhancing ideas that will help you spice up your everyday dishes and your special occasions, too.

- Use fresh herbs whenever possible. Use a mortar and pestle to grind them for the freshest and fullest flavor.
- Grate fresh ginger with a flat, sheet-type grater. Use a food processor to grate fresh horseradish—fresh packs a lot more punch than the salted, bottled kind.
- Add dried herbs such as thyme, rosemary and marjoram to dishes for a more pungent flavor, but use them sparingly.
- Use citrus zest, the colored part of the peel without the pit. It holds the true flavor of the fruit. Grate it with a flat, sheet-type grater or remove it with a vegetable peeler and cut the pieces into thin strips.
- Toast seeds, nuts and whole spices to bring out their full flavor. Cook them in a dry skillet over moderate heat or on a baking sheet in a 400-degree Fahrenheit oven.
- Roasting vegetables in a hot oven will caramelize their natural sugars and bring out their full flavor. You can achieve this without any oil!

- Use vinegar or citrus juice for a wonderful flavor-enhancer, but add it at the last moment. Vinegar is great on vegetables such as greens, and citrus works well on fruits such as melons. Either is great with fish.
- Use dry mustard for a zesty flavor in cooking or mix it with water to make a very sharp condiment.
- For a little more "bite" to your dishes, add fresh hot peppers. Remove the membrane and the seeds before finely chopping. And remember: a small amount goes a long way!
- Some vegetables and fruits, such as mushrooms, tomatoes, chili peppers, cherries, cranberries and currants, have a more intense flavor when dried than when fresh. Use them when you want a burst of flavor. Plus, there's an added bonus: when they're soaked in water and reconstituted, you can use the flavored water in cooking.
- Add dill to chicken, tuna or egg salad.
- Consider a flavored hummus (garlic, dill, lemon) in lieu of mayonnaise.
- Roast a whole clove of garlic in the oven and use the cooked garlic on bread instead of butter. (You may want to chase it down with parsley to neutralize your breath.)

CHAPTER 10
Living Skinny in Fat Genes™ (Putting It All Together: Your Action Plan)

So how does it all happen? The moment you've all been waiting for! Well, once we have set our eyes on the prize and set our goals (a new wardrobe), we have to implement it. First, we start with our caloric intake needs (budget) and then we'll have to break it down into numbers of servings from each food group (knowing portion sizes).

HOW MANY SERVINGS DO YOU NEED?

When people look at MyPyramid.gov, they have no idea how many **actual** servings they need as an INDIVIDUAL (nor do they know the serving sizes). What one ends up with is a total amount (quantity) needed in a day—which can be rather confusing when it comes to real food choices! As I often explain to my clients, think of it like money in your wallet: you have some singles, fives, tens, twenties, fifties, and if you're lucky, a few hundreds. Imagine that every day you MUST spend whatever is in your wallet. This is how I recommend that people think about their numbers of servings each day.

I have analyzed thousands of food journals personally. Some of the most useful information I can share with my clients is that when we look at the total number of calories consumed each day, there are often great fluctuations on a daily basis (from a few hundred to over a thousand calories).

For example, let's say that my daily caloric intake for five days was as follows: 1,500; 2,500; 1,200; 2,000; 1,800. Can you see that there is a jump in calories—both up and down? The problem here would be those thrifty genes that we have, which slow down when calories are scarce and store extra fat when calories are plentiful. So, in trying to achieve your weight loss and even maintenance, you need to try to achieve daily caloric intakes which are at the same level. If you are off by one hundred calories, it's not a big deal, but if it is more than 250 calories each day, you could be sabotaging your efforts.

Once you get in the swing of things, it will feel natural and comfortable—the way your jeans feel after you've worn them for a while (you know how they can feel right out of the dryer… then by the end of the day… ahhhhh).

The guide below will help you to understand the calorie levels and numbers of servings from each of the food groups. Use fats, oils and sweets sparingly.

SERVINGS OF FOOD GROUPS PER CALORIE LEVEL

Daily Recommended Calorie Intake	1200 kcal	1400 kcal	1600 kcal	1800 kcal	2000 kcal	2200 Kcal	2400 kcal	2600 kcal	2800 kcal
Grains	4	5	5	6	7	8	9	10	11
Vegetables	3	3	4	4.5	4.5	6	6	6	6.5
Fruits	2	2.5	2.5	2.5	4	4	4	4	4.5
Dairy	3	3	3	3	3	3	3	3	3
Meat, Poultry, Fish, Eggs, Beans, Nuts, Seeds	2	2	2	2	2	2	2	3	3
Daily Totals	3oz	4oz	5oz	6oz	6oz	7oz	8oz	9oz	10oz

For those who may have larger caloric needs, check out MyPyramid.gov to calculate your numbers of servings from each of the food groups.

SERVING SIZES

Try to measure your servings whenever possible and look at food labels. Below I list the serving sizes for each of the food groups. My motto is that all foods can fit! When possible, fresh is best! Many people assume that a package is a serving. Not the case! Have you ever bought a package of underwear or socks? You need to read the label and determine the "serving size." Whether you decide to eat the entire package is your choice. However, if you want to know how to count or categorize those foodstuffs into the number of portions you need in the day, be a savvy label reader! Just as when you are buying clothes, you need to make sure the number on the label (like the price of jeans) fits your budget! You need to know what really constitutes a serving.

Grains: Bread, Rice, Cereal and Pasta

- 1 slice of bread
- ½ cup of *cooked* pasta, rice, kasha, wheat berries, quinoa, etc.
- 1 tortilla (as long as it has fewer than 150 calories)
- ½ bagel or English muffin (unless it's the 100-calorie variety)
- 1 oz dry cereal (which would be indicated by cup serving on the food label)
- ½ c. hot cereal
- 1 4-inch-diameter pancake
- 1 small waffle
- 1 small muffin (2.5-inch diameter)
- 2 cups air-popped popcorn
- 1 serving of pretzels or baked chips (refer to food label)

- 1 2-inch square of angel food cake
- 1 "sheet" of graham crackers
- 100-calorie snack pack (crackers, cookies, snack chips)

It would be preferable that you consume as many whole-grain and unprocessed products as possible, but let's face it—everything in this category is "processed" and does not resemble the food as its ingredients are found in nature. In addition to carbohydrates, these foods contain amino acids (the building blocks of protein), fiber, vitamins and minerals. Try to find grains that have at least 4 grams of fiber per serving (Note: White or brown rice often does not have much fiber.)

Vegetables
- ½ cup of cooked or raw vegetables
- 1 cup of tightly packed leafy greens
- 8-10 baby carrots
- 6 ounces of tomato or vegetable juice
- 1 small baked potato (While some people consider this a starch, it is technically a vegetable. I once saw an ad for potatoes that showed a potato half dipped in green paint with a message that read, "What else do we have to do to prove to you that a potato is a vegetable?")
- 1 ear of corn
- 1 oz dried vegetables
- 1 cup of vegetable soup (at last ½ cup veggies and the rest broth)

Once again, these foods contain fiber, phytonutrients (the

pigments in plants that have added health benefits), amino acids (the building blocks of protein), carbohydrates, vitamins, and minerals. Try to choose greens that are dark or diverse in color. Iceberg lettuce is not poison, but it's not as nutrient-rich as other vegetables. Our diets simply do NOT have enough veggies. Not only do the statistics show that, but I can safely say while I have not kept stats on my entire clients' nutrient analyses, I can tell you this was the most common theme. Try to avoid drowning your veggies in too much fat or eating them fried!

Fruits

- 1 medium whole fruit (including bananas)
- ½ cup berries, grapes or melon (diced)
- 1 melon wedge
- 6 ounces of fruit juice
- ¼ cup dried fruit (raisins)
- ½ cup of apple sauce or fruit cup

This group contains fiber, water, vitamins, minerals, phyto-nutrients, carbohydrates, water, and lots of flavor!

Milk/Dairy

- 1 cup (8 ounces) of milk or yogurt (preferably skim/fat-free or 1%—the difference is the saturated-fat content)
- ½ cup of cottage cheese
- 1 ounce of cheese (a 1 inch x 1 inch cube, 1 string cheese, 1 cold-cut slice)
- ¼ cup of frozen yogurt or ice cream (okay, this really is grasping at straws)
- ½ cup of Jell-O pudding made with skim milk

This group contains vitamins, minerals, carbohydrates, sometimes fat, and is an excellent source of protein! The lower the fat content of your dairy product, the better your health outcome! Research has shown that consuming calcium and vitamin D in dairy products can be effective for weight loss!

Meat, Poultry, Fish, Beans, Seeds, Eggs, Nuts, and Nut Butters

- 1 egg (whole is fine)
- 2 tablespoons of nut butter
- ½ cup of cooked beans or legumes
- 1 ounce of cold-cuts
- 1 ounce of tofu
- nuts & seeds vary by the specific item (but ~ ¼ cup)
- 3-ounce portions of meat, chicken, fish, turkey, etc. (the size of the palm of your hand without fingers, or a deck of card)

This group contains vitamins, minerals, protein and in some instances fat. The leaner the meat, the better your health outcome. For the most part, the portions listed above are what one ounce of protein will be. Use your daily protein budget efficiently.

FATS, OILS, AND CONDIMENTS

I purposely do not tell you that you must eat a certain number of servings from this food group because I am assuming that fats will be used in the cooking process. It is up to you whether or not you want to drown your salad in dressing. It's your pants that you're trying to fit into. You have to answer to yourself. My recommendation is that you use as little fat as possible, so if you want to eat a piece of cake at a party later on, you just don't have to worry about the extra calories! It is simply about calories and trade-offs.

PUTTING IT ALL TOGETHER

Consider the numbers of servings you can have as money in your wallet that you must spend every day. When you consider eating, try thinking about consuming foods in this pattern:

Here is Felicia's Meal Plan Worksheet with examples of how to make all foods fit into the different calorie levels—without feeling deprived or hungry!

Felicia's Meal Plan Worksheet
Calorie Level _____

Number of
Servings   Food Group

_____   Grains (try to choose high-fiber foods): bread (1 sl), rice (½ c), cereal (1 oz), pasta (½ c), whole grains

_____   Fruits: 1 medium, 6 oz juice, ½ cup sauce/cocktail, ¼ cup dried

_____   Vegetables: 6 oz juice, ½ c. cooked/chopped, 1 cup tightly packed leafy greens

_____   Dairy: Fluid milk/yogurt (8 oz/1 c), cheese (1 oz), cottage cheese (½ c)

_____ = ____oz (total) Protein: Meat, Poultry, Fish, Eggs

(1=1 oz), Nuts/Seeds (¼ c = 1 oz), Beans/Legumes (½ c = 1 oz), Nut Butter (2 tbs = 1 oz)

Breakfast
  Snack 1
Lunch
  Snack 2
Dinner
  Snack 3

Here is an example of an 1,800-calorie meal plan:

# Servings/day	Food Group
6	Grains: Bread, Rice, Cereal, Pasta
2.5	Fruits
5	Vegetables
3	Dairy
2: 6oz daily total	Meat, Poultry, Fish, Eggs, Beans, Nuts, Seeds

Sample Eating Pattern	Actual Menu Idea
Breakfast 1 Grain 1 Fruit 1 Dairy	**Breakfast** 1/3 cup All-Bran Bran Buds cereal 1 banana 4 ounces vanilla Greek yogurt 0% Fat
Snack 1 1 Fruit	**Snack 1** Apple

Lunch 2 Grains 2 Vegetables 1 Dairy 3 ounces meat	**Lunch** 2 slices whole-grain, high-fiber bread 3 ounces tuna w/lemon juice & dill, lettuce & tomato (on sandwich), 1 side salad w/veggies, 1 ounce shredded cheese on salad, 2 tbs salad dressing of choice
Snack 2 1 Grain	**Snack 2** 2 cups of air-popped popcorn
Dinner 2 Grains 2.5 Vegetables 3 ounces meat	**Dinner** 1 cup of couscous 1.5 cups of grilled vegetables 3 ounces herb-roasted chicken breast
Snack 3 1 Dairy	**Snack 3** 1 cup Jell-O fat-free (not sugar-free) vanilla or chocolate pudding

An important, underlying factor to remember is that the slower you shed those pounds, the more likely you will be to maintain the weight loss over time and stay in your new skinny genes. It means carefully selecting food on a daily basis and making physical activity part of your rituals (just like brushing your teeth). Taking one day at time and not being your biggest critic is the best way to finally get into those skinny genes!

CHAPTER 11

Let's Go Shopping– Recipes, Shopping Lists, Tips

● ●

This chapter contains my favorite foods lists—snacking, eating on the run (especially for the traveler), shopping lists, tips and recipes. There will be suggestions and recommendations by food groups, staple items to have on hand, snacks you can leave in your handbag, car or office to help you during a moment of hunger. This section will teach you how to read food labels so that you know how to get directly to the important information that you need in order to make better choices about what you put in your mouth. There will be "staples" (like your favorite belt to go with all your jeans) to keep on hand.

Clients are often surprised when I let them know what they "can" and "cannot" eat. In all fairness, I try to show people how to make better food choices. However, it would be unrealistic for me to assume that you grow and cook your own food. It would be nice, but it's not realistic. As a practitioner, I have to take into account those food items that are accessible and available to those seeking my advice. If you are going to be successful at losing the weight, keeping it off for good, and maintaining some changed behavior, then we have to work with what you will actually DO!

If you could prepare most of your own food and minimize the amount of packaged and processed food, you would probably save yourself money and better control the calories, fat and sodium in your food. Hopefully, you can be more honest with yourself when you dole out your portions of foods as well! If you cheat, you only cheat yourself!

ARE YOU A SAVVY LABEL READER?

You know how to find the size and price of a garment of clothing, but how good are you at eyeballing the important information on a food label? Let's explore the Nutrition Facts Panel and ingredient list. The ingredient list is the easiest to explain— which basically is a list of the ingredients found in a product, listed in the order in which they appear by volume from greatest amount to least amount (like looking at the thread count in your blouse—how much is cotton, silk, polyester, etc.). If you have food allergies or know that certain ingredients may trigger headaches, rashes, upset stomach, etc., you know that reviewing this list is essential to making sure you do not get sick.

For the rest of us, we all have our own personal list of things we are trying to avoid. For me, it is all about avoiding any sugar substitutes or artificial sweeteners: sucralose, saccharine, acesulfame potassium, aspartame, stevia, and sugar alcohols (malitol, sorbitol, erythritol, xylitol). I must admit, I am a super taster—my tongue can sense the presence of these ingredients in a food product. With the exception of chewing gum, the taste of the food item in which this is hiding can really send an undesirable sensory message to my brain. I remember taking a taste test in the classroom at Teachers College, where our professor handed out little paper strips that resembled pH strips. If you placed one on your tongue and you had no sensation, you were not a supertaster. If you experienced a bitter taste in your mouth—well, you just won the prize!

From a healthcare provider perspective, as someone who has worked with people struggling with weight, I have observed the surplus of sugar substitutes and artificial sweeteners that my clients consume. I would have people coming into my office who were more than 100 pounds overweight and who drank liters of "diet" soft drinks every day. When I was a student, we learned to be skeptical about people's accuracy of food reporting, but I did observe a trend that made me take a step back and look at satiety and digestion. If I eat or drink something that tastes "sweet," my tongue sends a message to the hypothalamus, which may "glucosense" that something "sweet" is coming down the pipes. So our body is anxiously waiting what it assumes are carbohydrates. The digestive system starts ramping up the system to prepare for its work to be done (like the parts in a mechanical car wash), which means that our lovely nervous system communicates a message that enzymes, bile acids and bicarb better get ready to receive this bolus. It may very well include the production and release of insulin from the pancreas. Research is still being conducted to understand this better.

Insulin serves as a lock-and-key mechanism to move glucose or fat into a cell, so its production is not necessarily dose-responsive, meaning it will be created, but not in the quantity to match the precise amount of carbohydrates it will need to process. So what happens is that we have insulin circulating in our blood stream, with the mission of escorting glucose into the cells for energy, but with the absence of added glucose, insulin will deposit fat into fat cells. Plain and simple. We have the ability to store an infinite amount of fat in our fat cells and our body does it rather well. The human body is an amazing "machine" made up of chemical and electrical reactions that try to maintain a level of homeostasis. This means that amounts of glucose, fat, amino acids, the acid-base balance, calcium, sodium, white blood cells, red blood cells, various hormones, etc., are all tightly regulated to yield certain "values" within a range.

Have you ever wondered about having a fever when you are sick? It is thought that a high fever will destroy any bacteria or viruses in the body. What makes elevated body temperature so dangerous—and this can be seen with heat stroke—is that proteins and enzymes in the body "denature," making them lose their shape, setting off a series of reactions that include the shift in the bloodstream's acid-base balance, fluid balance and decreased ability to regulate body processes. If your blood is too acidic or too basic, you will die.

What do YOU need to know about the information on the Nutrition Facts Panel? Well, let's start at the top and work our way down. The first line will read SERVING SIZE, which tells you what the standardized portion for this item is—usually in cups or ounces (it usually adheres to USDA food standardization). It will also tell you the NUMBER OF SERVINGS in the package (which means, for more than one serving—you must multiply the number of servings PER PACKAGE by the nutrition information to find out how much is in the whole package). The next important number is CALORIES—this is per serving of the food item. Calories represent the amount of energy you get from one serving of the food.

INGREDIENTS WE NEED TO CONSUME LESS

This is followed by CALORIES FROM FAT—defining fat content by calories—and in my opinion, not as important as the next few lines. TOTAL FAT, SATURATED FAT, TRANS FAT— now these you want to keep as low as possible. It is challenging to make a recommendation never to eat foods with a certain amount of grams of fat in each serving, because it is about total intake for the day—not just in one food item. For example, nuts have fat—mostly good fats, but they do have fats—so it would be incorrect to state that if you see X quantity of fat on a label, don't eat that food.

Next on the list of information is CHOLESTEROL and SODIUM. Dietary intake of CHOLESTEROL does not increase your serum cholesterol levels; whereas SATURATED and TRANS FAT can impact those numbers. Foods of plant origin do not contain cholesterol. Foods derived from animals do contain cholesterol. You should consider consuming no more than 300 mg of cholesterol each day. Three ounces of chicken breast meat only has 75 milligrams of cholesterol; three ounces of steak has 65 milligrams of cholesterol, three ounces of salmon contains 54 milligrams of cholesterol.

SODIUM intake should be under 2,400 mg per day for most Americans. The latest U.S. Dietary Guidelines suggest 1,500 mg each day. If you have high blood pressure, take certain medications which are affected by sodium, or are sodium sensitive (you retain water after eating salty foods), then you would be wise to pay attention to this value on the label. Sodium, as a mineral, is naturally occurring in some foods. However over 75 percent of sodium in our diets comes from processed and package foods. What is the equivalent of 2,400 mg of sodium? Almost one teaspoon of table salt or two tablespoons of soy sauce.

Sodium is essential in the diet because it plays a role in nerve transmission, maintaining fluid balance, and influencing muscle contraction and relaxation in the body.

The reason we need to consume less of these nutrients is that high consumption rates are correlated with heart disease, obesity, high cholesterol, high blood pressure and certain cancers.

WHAT ELSE IS LEFT?

CARBOHYDRATES are next—and often I find that many people do not know how many grams of carbohydrates they need in a day. I'm so bad with numbers, I can't think of my foods as grams of every ingredient—so why should you? This value can be misleading, and truly, it is best suited for diabetics who need to know how many grams of carbohydrates they are eating, so they can moderate their exogenous insulin dosing.

My favorite "f" word—FIBER. Remember, some foods do not have any fiber (like a packet of tuna), so when you can choose foods that have a high amount of fiber (hint, hint—the grain group), this number can be quite helpful! If by chance, SOLUBLE or INSOLUBLE FIBER is specified, it really doesn't matter for general nutrition and weight-loss purposes. It's just more numbers to confuse you. Our bodies are not like those digital coin sorters that keep track of the total amount going in! SUGAR is the other word, that demon that is really part of total carbohydrates. It is confusing in that it does not represent added sugars and it includes naturally occurring sugars. If you notice, total grams of CARBOHYDRATES are often identical to the total grams of SUGARS. Our brains rely on carbohydrates, and remember—we have limited storage capacity, so we must ingest it throughout the day.

PROTEIN is also listed on the label. Remember, some foods are inherently high in protein (like nuts) whereas others (like fruits) are not. So don't look for Orange Juice to be a good source of protein. Likewise, don't expect a chicken breast to be a good source of fiber! We only need a limited amount each day—so don't over consume it!

DAILY VALUES IN PERCENTAGES

I sat in on a focus group in Washington, D.C., several years ago to speak about this very topic. As a clinician who tries to help make the science easy for the consumer, I think this entire food column is a waste and is confusing. Do you know what it represents? The percent of nutrients this one food item has relative to the daily caloric intake needs based upon a 2,000-calorie/day diet. Guess what? Most people don't need 2,000 calories, so what is the point of those percentage values? Really, what information is useful to an individual? Percentage daily value does not help one to figure out how this food really fits into their daily calorie budget (unless they've got the Excel spreadsheet and a laptop nearby). So, my advice to you is to ignore it, just like I do.

While keeping track of your caloric intake can be an essential part of your weight loss and maintenance, turning you into a savant is not the goal here; it's unrealistic and it does not encourage you to think about your relationship with food and to "normalize" eating. I want you to stop being an obsessive/compulsive number person who worries about every number on a food label, and learn to choose foods by the numbers of servings from the various food groups and understand what an appropriate portion is for each food group/category.

GRAB 'N GO FOOD IDEAS
- Yogurt shakes (pre-packaged)
- Mini snack bags of baked potato chips, pretzels, popcorn, baked tortilla chips, graham crackers, whole-grain crackers

- Apple sauce
- Fruit cups
- 1%-fat cottage cheese cups
- String cheese (2%)
- Soup cups
- Rice & bean cups
- Peanut butter & jelly sandwiches
- Raisin or Craisin boxes
- Dried fruits/veggies
- Granola bars
- Nuts such as almonds, walnuts, etc. (avoid salted)
- Baked chips (or Popchips)

IDEAS FOR HEALTHFUL SNACKS FOR EATING ON THE RUN

Fruits—fresh, dried, frozen, canned, packaged

- Apples
- Bananas
- Cherries
- FrozFruit (like a Popsicle, but doesn't have added sugar, so it's healthier)
- Grapes
- Kiwi (sometimes available precut)
- Mangoes (sometimes available precut)
- Oranges/Tangerines/Clementines/Grapefruit
- Pears
- Papayas (sometimes available precut)
- Peaches and plums (in summer)
- Raisins and other dried fruit (such as apricots, dates, and figs)

- Vegetables
- Carrots (pre-peeled and washed are convenient)
- Celery
- Peppers—sliced red and green peppers
- Tomatoes (small tomatoes like cherry or grape tomatoes are easy to snack on; all tomatoes are best in late summer)

Nuts are nutritious but high in fat, so only eat a small amount.

- Mixed nuts with raisins
- Peanuts in shells
- Peanut butter (makes a great dip for fruits, such as apples, or vegetables such as carrots)
- Other
- Hard-boiled eggs
- Whole-grain bread
- Popcorn (if possible, pop your own, and don't add fat)
- Pretzels
- Rice cakes (look for the flavored types)
- Small yogurts (especially the Greek style)
- Edamame (dried, boiled/steamed)

GROCERY LIST FOR PEOPLE ON THE GO

This list assumes you have access to hot water and/or a microwave for certain items.

Fruits
- Obtain fresh when you can.
- Dried fruits of your choice. Make sure dried fruits do not have added sugar.
- Consider Sunsweet individually wrapped plums (yum)

- Dehydrated fruits:
- www.justtomatoes.com/ (this has been a favorite brand of mine even before I became an RD!)
- www.brothersallnatural.com/ (a new favorite!)
- www.edenfoods.com/store/index.php?cPath=75_76
- www.sensiblefoods.com/
- Fruit juice counts, but it's loaded with extra calories & usually has no fiber.

Vegetables
- www.justtomatoes.com/ (this has been a favorite brand of mine even before I became an RD!)
- www.brothersallnatural.com/ (a new favorite!)
- www.edenfoods.com/store/index.php?cPath=75_76
- www.sensiblefoods.com/
- Veggie juice counts, V8 or tomato, too
- Try to focus on eating fresh food when you can

Dairy
- Cheese (there are shelf-stable varieties in all supermarkets—they're the cheeses that are NOT in the refrigerator case).
- Shelf-stable milk, rice milk, soymilk in small packaging (can go in your suitcase)
- Many individually wrapped cheeses can be out of refrigeration for several hours.

Protein
- Nuts and seeds are always great. Try to limit sodium when you can.
- www.edenfoods.com/store/index.php?cPath=75_76

Tuna, chicken & salmon now come in small cups & foil pouches:

- Chicken of the Sea has shelf-stable pouches with tuna, salmon & shrimp
- Starkist also has tuna & salmon (including seasoned filets): www.starkist.com/template .asp?section=products/index.html
- Tyson Chicken www.tyson.com/recipes/Product/ ViewProduct.aspx?id=101

These are options if you do not have access to prepared protein foods:

- Dried soybeans are also great to take along
- www.seapointfarms.com/products.asp?cat=47& hierarchy=0 (these are a personal favorite of mine)
- Peanut butter... natural is my preference... Justin's Nut Butters come in individual squeeze packs www.justinsnutbutter.com/)
- Hummus is also great (some brands have individual containers)
- 100-calorie nut packs
- Cocoa-dusted almonds

Grains

- Uncle Ben's Ready Rice packets
- Minute Rice Ready to Serve cups
- Kashi Whole-Grain Pilaf
- Whole-grain crackers

Other shelf-stable "meals"/snacks

- www.carringtonfarms.com/products.cfm?product= %20Flax-Paks (You can sprinkle this into anything.)

- Annie Chun's soups/rice/noodle dishes: www.anniechuns.com
- My new favorite: www.crystalnoodle.com/html/
- Thai Kitchen: www.thaikitchen.com/
- St. Dalfour Gourmet on the Go: www.shopping.com/ -st.+dalfour+gourmet+on+the+go
- Kitchens of India: www.kitchensofindia.com/ (Note: there are other brands of shelf-stable Indian food that is pre-cooked & just needs to be warmed up.)
- Carman's Muesli Bars: www.carmansfinefoods.com.au/
- Kind Fruit & Nut Bars: www.kindsnacks.com
- Lära Bars: www.larabar.com
- Mary's Gone Crackers: www.marysgonecrackers.com/
- There are several brands of soup/rice/cous-cous instant cups. Some have beans, too!

Cereals:

- Any brand you like that has at least 3 grams of fiber per serving
- Kashi
- Kellogg's All-Bran Products (Bran Buds are my favorite)
- General Mills Fiber One products
- Whole Foods 365 Organic Instant Oatmeal
- Post Shredded Wheat

Vending Machine Options

Let's face it—sometimes you find yourself really hungry, your blood sugar levels may be dropping and you need a quick nibble. The only food around may come out of a vending machine. In general, vending machines do not always have the better choices—but there certainly are healthy options if you know what to look for. (Try to aim for less than 200 calories— although they are seldom displayed).

- Any baked snack chip—potato chips, pretzels, crackers, tortilla chips, cheese puffs
- Packs of nuts (hopefully dry roasted)/unsalted trail mix
- Cereal or granola bar
- Snack-size pack of cookies: Fig Newtons, graham crackers, or other baked treat
- Cereal box
- Small chocolate bar—simple ones like York Peppermint Patty, Hershey Bar, M&Ms

Dress-Up Jeans—Dining Out

You can go out to eat and not throw all your efforts in the old-clothes bin if you plan ahead and think of eating as a necessary part of life. If every time you go out to eat your mind thinks it's a special occasion and you can have whatever you want, you will be sabotaging yourself—because most people are eating more and more meals away from home. The first tip is to make sure there are items that you can eat at the restaurant you are going to. Treat food as if you were allergic to an ingredient, and by this I mean, don't go to a restaurant where absolutely everything is fried, when you are trying to avoid fried foods, for example. The second tip: don't arrive famished. Make sure you had something to snack on. When you are overhungry, you will not make the best food choices and will probably overeat (especially if you eat quickly). Go easy on the alcohol—the caloric value of alcohol is closer to fat than carbohydrates or protein. Go easy on the booze because the extra calories can add up rather quickly. Here are some healthy options:

- Vegetarian pizza
- Vegetable-based soups (gazpacho)
- Consommé
- Vegetable or fruit plate
- Salad with dressing on the side
- Steamed, grilled or roasted vegetables
- Baked potatoes (all accoutrements on the side)
- Grilled chicken, fish
- Lean meat (filet mignon), pork (yes, it's the other white meat)
- Vegetable patties
- Regular size burgers (the small ones)
- Yogurt shakes (low-fat or fat-free yogurt)
- Sandwiches (skip the mayo or have it on the side) on wheat, rye, or whole-grain breads with mustard, salsa, or low-fat mayo
- Fresh fruit, sorbet, or angel food cake
- Cappuccino (skim or low-fat milk)
- Tortilla wraps (skip sour cream)

Tips for ordering:
- Order à la carte (my favorite)
- Order soup and salad in lieu of a full meal (order one extra appetizer as an entrée)
- Order all dressing & sauces on the side

- Order a meal as if you were eating at home
- Move bread or chips to the other side of the table (if you think you will overeat them)
- Avoid buffets (it's not about the value)
- Pay attention to alcohol and soft-drink consumption

Words to look for when ordering food:

- Au jus (cooked in its own juice)
- Baked
- Braised
- Broiled
- Marinara
- Primavera (vegetables)
- Poached
- Roasted
- Steamed
- Stir-fried (ask them to go light on the oil)
- Vinaigrette

Words to avoid when ordering food:

- Alfredo
- Au gratin
- Cheese sauce
- Béarnaise
- Breaded
- Beurre blanc
- Buttered
- Creamed
- Crispy
- Double crust

- En croûte
- Fried: Deep, French, pan
- Pastry
- Prime
- Rich
- Sautéed
- Scalloped
- White sauces

I'm a big fan of grab 'n go foods. The pre-packaged smoothies (with and without dairy) are great—just stick a straw in and drink away! Some other favorite foods:

- Kind Fruit+Nut bars
- Fat-free or low-fat yogurt
- 3 oz white tuna in water in foil packets
- Lara bars
- Kashi bars
- String cheese (2% fat)
- Edamame
- Kraft South Beach Bars
- Odwalla bars and beverages
- Hard-boiled eggs
- Laughing Cow Low-Fat Cheese
- Jamba Juice Smoothies
- Nuts—dry roasted or raw
- Seeds—dry roasted or raw

Recipe Modification

Some people simply cannot fathom changing their aunt's favorite recipe. For me, it's about making items healthier!

Original Ingredient	Substitution Suggestion
Butter, margarine, shortening or lard	1/4 less liquid oil or solid fat called for in the recipe
Shortening, butter, or oil in baking	Applesauce or prune puree for half of the butter, shortening or oil. Reduce baking time by 25%
Butter, shortening, margarine, or oil to prevent sticking , sauté or stir-fry.	Cooking spray, water, broth or nonstick pans
Whole milk, half and half or evaporated milk	Skim or low-fat milk
Full-fat cream cheese	Low-fat or nonfat cream cheese, Neufchâtel or low-fat cottage cheese pureed until smooth.
Full-fat sour cream, cottage cheese or ricotta cheese	Nonfat or reduced fat sour cream, fat-free plain yogurt, part-skim ricotta
Cream Whipping cream	Evaporated skim milk Nonfat whipped topping or cream
Eggs	Egg whites (2 egg whites for each egg) or 1/2 cup egg substitute per egg
Whole-fat cheese	Reduced-fat cheese, but add it at the end of the baking time or use part-skim mozzarella
Regular mayonnaise or salad dressing	Low-fat, reduced or nonfat mayonnaise, hummus or salad dressing. I like to use hummus in place of mayo for tuna or chicken salad.

For great, nutritious recipes go to www.aicr.org. You can sign up for free weekly recipes by e-mail. Here's a great chicken dish you can try with some veggies:

Moroccan Chicken with Tomatoes and Honey

This unpretentious chicken and tomato dish is enlivened by mysterious notes of cinnamon and ginger.

> ¼ tsp. ground turmeric or saffron threads
>
> 2 Tbsp. extra virgin olive oil
>
> 1 large onion, finely chopped
>
> 2 medium (1½ lb.) skinless chicken breasts, with ribs, halved
>
> 2½ lbs. ripe plum tomatoes, peeled, seeded and chopped (see note)
>
> 1 tsp. ground cinnamon
>
> 1 tsp. ground ginger
>
> 3 Tbsp. honey
>
> 1 tsp. salt
>
> 4 cups cooked hot couscous

1. If using saffron, place in small bowl and add 2 tablespoons hot water. Let sit until saffron is dissolved, about 20 minutes, before using.

2. Heat oil in large Dutch oven or deep pan over medium-high heat. Sauté onion until golden, about

6 minutes. Remove with slotted spoon and transfer to plate.

3. Add chicken and sauté, turning frequently, until browned on all sides, about 8 minutes. Remove chicken to plate and set aside.

4. Add ½ cup water to pan, scraping bottom with a wooden spoon to loosen all browned bits. Add tomatoes and cook until softened, about 8 minutes. Stir in turmeric (or saffron), cinnamon, ginger, honey and salt to taste. Return chicken and onion to pot. Cover tightly and gently simmer until chicken is very tender, about 50 minutes.

5. Serve ladled over hot couscous.

Note: Three pounds (the equivalent of 48 ounces) canned peeled tomatoes, drained and chopped, may be substituted.

EAT MORE SPINACH

Popeye isn't the only one who knows that spinach is good for you. It is always listed among the "superfoods" that are loaded with ingredients that are good for you: vitamins A, B (thiamin, riboflavin, B6 and folate), C, E and K, magnesium, iron, phosphorous, zinc, selenium, manganese, lutein, alphalipoic acid (ALA), polyphenols, omega-3 fatty acids and dietary fiber. Do I have you convinced yet? Well, let me share a favorite recipe that can be prepared in advance and frozen until ready to use. I have served this as an appetizer and as a side dish. I usually have to double the recipe because everyone loves them!

Spinach Balls

2 packages of frozen chopped spinach, thawed and drained

2 cups of Pepperidge Farm Stuffing (or any small cut stuffing)—may use matzoh farfel (great way to use this recipe during Passover as well)

1 onion chopped

8 egg whites

½ cup melted butter

½ cup grated parmesan

¼ Tsp. nutmeg

1. Preheat the oven to 375 degrees.

2. Combine all ingredients in a large bowl.

3. Form into bite-sized balls and place on a cookie sheet or pan that has been coated with nonstick spray.

4. Bake for 20 minutes and serve (turn them gently halfway)

Yield: 36 spinach balls.

Note: The spinach balls can be frozen and placed in a container (separate the layers with wax paper or aluminum foil). Defrost 20 minutes before baking and then bake as above. Also, in lieu of rolling balls, you can bake this in a square, nonstick or Pyrex dish and cut into squares.

Remember, there are many holidays throughout the year. These are months which seem to be more dense with eating opportunities beyond your regular meals (Nov.–Jan.; May–Aug.)!

There is so much to be grateful for… plentiful food, friends, and good health! Instead of starting your diet on Monday—make better choices every day!

Hasselback Potatoes

Super easy to make—can even make them on the BBQ over the summer (wrap each potato in foil).

> Take baking potatoes (any type—just not small potatoes)—can use red skin or white skin potatoes (one/person)
> Salt as needed
> Olive oil as needed

1. Preheat oven to 450 degrees. Place each potato between the handle of two wooden spoons (or chopsticks). Carefully cut (to the spoon or chopstick) with a sharp knife, into the potato. Make additional cuts ¼ inch (or smaller) apart.

2. Brush w/olive oil and sprinkle with salt. You may take dried garlic slices or fresh cloves and place in each slit (optional). Bake for one hour in the oven. (I prefer to put it on top of parchment, so it doesn't stick). Baste with the oil during the hour.

3. You may add herbs to taste.

"Kettle" Cauliflower

Take 1 large head of cauliflower and cut into small pieces

In a bowl mix the following:

> 8 tbs oil (olive may be too strong in flavor—I use blended
> oil or Malaysian Palm Oil)
> ½ tsp paprika
> ½ tsp tumeric
> ¼ tsp garlic powder
> ¼ tsp onion powder
> 1 tsp salt
> 2 tsp sugar

1. Preheat the oven to 450 degrees.

2. Coat the cauliflower with the oil and seasonings.
   Place on a baking sheet that is lined with parchment
   paper. Cook for 30 minutes. Turn the mixture 1–2
   times during the baking process.

Note: The cauliflower reduces in volume during the cooking.

Felicia's New Orleans-Style Jammin' Jambalaya

This recipe was given to me by a college acquaintance. I have
modified it to fit many diverse people's needs. It can be made
strictly vegetarian, it can be made without shellfish or red meat,
or without sausage at all. The preparation is pretty much the

same (except for the roux—which I have found is unnecessary). I have cooked it with and without the roux and prefer the recipe without the roux. It can be low in fat, cholesterol and sodium. Note: All meats are optional and can be made vegetarian or modified as you would like.

1 lb chicken breast

1 lb sausage (pork, turkey or vegetarian)

1 lb peeled shrimp (optional)

4 medium size onions

1 green pepper

1 red pepper

3 cloves of garlic

1 can Rotelle tomatoes—a brand name for canned, seasoned tomatoes & peppers & chiles. You may also use Italian/Mexican-style tomatoes

1 cup rice (Uncle Ben's© or Carolina)

2½ cups of water

Cayenne Pepper to taste

¼ tsp. McIlhenny Co. Tabasco Pepper Sauce

Cut chicken & sausage into small pieces

Dice the onions, garlic & peppers

1. In a skillet, cook the chicken & sausage (& shrimp)

2. Add onions, garlic & peppers

3. Put the above into a large pot; add tomatoes, rice, water & cayenne pepper

4. Cover & cook on low heat for 30 minutes (maybe longer, the mixture should be "dry" not soupy). This may also be made in a large or disposable roasting pan—covered, and placed in the oven (at 375°) for at least 45 minutes.

Yields dinner for 4 or side dish for 8.

Vegetarian Couscous Paella

Serves 4; 1¼ cups per serving

Vegetable oil spray

1 small red onion

2 tsp minced garlic

1½ cups vegetable or chicken broth

1 cup (8 oz) baby lima beans (frozen or canned)

1 cup (8 oz) baby sweet peas

¼ tsp salt

½ tsp ground tumeric

$1/_8$ tsp ground red (cayenne) pepper

1 cup dry couscous

1 medium tomato (or 1 small can chopped tomatoes)

¼ cup fresh cilantro or parsley

1. Spray a large saucepan or Dutch oven with vegetable oil spray.

2. Place over medium-high heat.

3. Add onion & garlic and cook until onion is tender (about 5 minutes).

4. Add broth, lima beans, peas, salt, tumeric and pepper.

5. Bring to a boil over high heat.

6. Reduce heat, cover & simmer 10 minutes or until lima beans are tender.

7. Remove from heat and stir in uncooked couscous, tomato, and cilantro.

8. Cover & let stand 5 minutes.

Red & Black Bean Salad

1 can black beans (15 oz)

1 can kidney beans (15 oz)

1 can Mexicorn (corn w/green peppers) (11 oz)

3 green onions (scallions) / ½ cup copped

3 tbs extra virgin olive oil

3 tbs red wine vinegar

½ tsp garlic powder

½ tsp cumin

¼ tsp salt (or to taste)

¼ tsp black pepper (or to taste)

1. Pour both cans of beans into a colander to drain; pour corn on top of the beans; rinse the vegetables w/cool water; drain well; pour vegetables into a 3-qt or larger bowl.

2. Finely chop the green onions using all of the white and the green tops to make ½ cup… add them to the bowl.

3. To make the dressing, pour the olive oil into a 2-cup glass measure; whisk in the vinegar, garlic powder, cumin, salt & black pepper.

4. Pour the mixture over the vegetables & stir until well mixed.

5. Serve at once or chill until ready to serve.

6. Serves 4 as a main dish; 8 as a side dish

Couscous Salad

1 bunch Romaine lettuce (or 1 package ready to use)

1 box Roasted Garlic Couscous (made ahead of time, use cold)

½ cup olive oil

½ cup lemon juice

1 cup grated Romano cheese

2 Cloves fresh chopped garlic

Croutons or Italian Panko crumbs (optional)

1. Let garlic sit in oil 6–8 hours before making salad (the longer the better)

2. Pour garlic oil on lettuce and mix until lightly wet

3. Pour lemon juice on lettuce and mix until wet (keep tasting at this point, sometimes adding more than ½ cup lemon)

4. Add grated cheese by the slowly mixing after each addition (taste as you go, may decrease or increase cheese)

5. Add cold couscous by slowly mixing after each addition

6. Croutons or Italian Panko crumbs can be used if desired

HINT: Mix salad 10 minutes before serving; it gets soggy quickly!

Tomato and Roasted Pepper Compote For Chicken or Swordfish

½ cup raisins

¼ cup white wine

2 red bell peppers (or buy roasted)

1 yellow bell pepper (or buy roasted)

medium tomatoes, peeled, seeded and diced

1½ cups leeks (round, white and light green parts only), washed

⅓ cup olive oil

1 cup chopped zucchini

1½ tsps. minced garlic

¼ cup pine nuts, lightly toasted

⅓ cup tightly packed basil, cut into thin strips

2 Tbsps. balsamic vinegar

¼ tsps. pepper

1. Combine the raisins and white wine in a small saucepan and bring to a simmer over medium heat. Remove immediately from the heat and set aside to plump.

2. Roast the peppers, remove skin. Cool. Skip this step if roasted peppers were purchased. Cut the peppers into 1-inch pieces. Place in a large bowl.

3. In a small sauté pan over low heat, cook the leeks in 2 tsps. of the olive oil until they are tender. Add to the peppers.

4. In the same pan, heat 2 tsps. of the olive oil and cook the zucchini over medium heat until softened but not limp. Combine with peppers and leeks.

5. In the same sauté pan, heat 2 tsps. of the olive oil and cook the tomatoes as desired. Add to the mixture.

6. Drain the raisins, discarding any remaining wine, and add to the compote along with the garlic, pine

nuts, basil, balsamic vinegar and remaining olive oil. Season as desired.

7. Either broil, bake, or grill swordfish or sauté boneless chicken breasts in olive oil. Serve compote on top.

Serves 4

Jalapeño Chicken

2 tsp ground cinnamon

2 tsp chili powder

1 tsp cumin powder

2 tsp salt

1 tsp black pepper

boneless, skinless chicken breasts

1 cup Healthy Request Chicken Broth

2 tbs honey

2 limes, juiced

1 jalapeño pepper, minced

1. Preheat oven to 450 degrees Fahrenheit. Lightly grease a medium baking sheet.

2. In a small bowl, mix the cinnamon, chili powder, cumin, salt, and pepper together. Rub the mixture onto the chicken and arrange the breast on the baking sheet.

3. In a medium saucepan, combine the chicken broth, honey, lime juice, and jalapeño. Cook over medium-high heat, stirring until the mixture thickens.

4. Cook chicken for about 15 minutes. Begin basting the chicken periodically with the broth mixture. Continue cooking for 30 minutes or until chicken is no longer pink and juices run clear.

Veggie Mac 'n Cheese

1 box whole grain elbow or spiral pasta

$^1/_2$ cup low sodium vegetable broth

1 cup fat-free half and half

$^1/_4$ tsp salt

$^1/_8$ tsp cayenne pepper

1 cup low fat shredded cheese (blend, cheddar, etc.)

$^1/_4$ cup grated parmesan cheese

1 16 oz. package of frozen broccoli (thawed)

1 12 oz. jar roasted bell peppers (in water), drained & diced

2 Tbsp. plain, whole wheat bread crumbs

1. Cook pasta to time, drain well in a colander.

2. In a medium saucepan, whisk together the broth, the half-and-half, salt and cayenne. Bring to a simmer for 1 to 2 minutes, or until thickened, whisking occasionally. Remove from the heat. Stir in the shredded cheese and parmesan until melted.

3. Meanwhile, preheat the oven to 350 degrees.

4. Place the cooked pasta into a casserole pan, stir in the broccoli, bell peppers and cheese sauce. Sprinkle with the bread crumbs. Bake for 25–30 minutes or until warmed through and golden brown on top.

Zydeco Green Beans

1 tsp olive oil

$^1/_2$ medium onion (or use $^1/_2$ cup frozen chopped)

$^1/_2$ medium green bell pepper chopped (or use $^1/_2$ cup frozen chopped)

1 medium rib of celery chopped

4 medium tomatoes diced (or 1 can diced)

1 cup (8 ounces) fresh green beans timed and cut into 1-inch pieces (or use frozen or canned)

1 cup water

$^1/_8$ tsp cayenne pepper

$^1/_4$ tsp red hot pepper sauce

1. In a medium saucepan, heat the oil over medium heat, cook the onion, bell pepper, and celery for 3–4 minutes, stirring occasionally.

2. Stir in the remaining ingredients. Reduce the heat and simmer for about 25 minutes.

Cucumbers with Dilled Yogurt

3 medium cucumbers, peeled and sliced into circles

1 small onion finely chopped

1 tsp sugar

$1/2$ cup fat-free plain Greek yogurt

1 tbs fresh dillweed (or dried)

1 tsp fresh lemon juice (or prepared)

$1/2$ tsp pepper

$1/4$ tsp salt

1. In a medium bowl, stir together the cucumbers and onions. Sprinkle in the sugar. Stir well. Cover and refrigerate for 1 hour. Drain excess fluid.

2. In a small bowl, whisk together the remaining ingredients. Add this to the cucumber/onion mixture, stir.

3. You can serve right away or let sit in the refrigerator.

Vinaigrette Coleslaw

8 oz. packaged shredded cabagge and carrot slaw mix
(~ 3 $1/2$ cups)

1 tsp canola oil

$1/2$ tsp celery seeds

$1/4$ tsp pepper

$^1/_8$ tsp salt

3 tbs cider vinegar

3 tbs sugar

In a small bowl, whisk the vinegar, sugar, salt, pepper, oil and celery seeds. Pour over the coleslaw mixture. Toss well. Serve immediately or refrigerate.

THE 12 MYTHS UNRIVETED

1. Eating/eliminating certain foods help you to lose weight

    a. Cutting carbohydrates helps you to lose weight

    b. Eating large quantities of protein foods will help you to lose weight

    c. Dairy foods make you fat (using soy in lieu of dairy)

    d. You can't eat nuts or red meat when trying to lose weight

    e. Sugar of all sorts (including fruit) & high fructose corn syrup make you fat

    f. All starches are bad for you

    g. Brown foods = whole grain = fiber

    h. Low-fat, fat-free or sugar-free foods = no calories

    i. All salads are healthy

    j. Artificial sweeteners can help you lose weight

    k. All fats are bad for you

2. Cutting calories below 1,200 kcal/day will help you to lose weight (each person is individual & unique).

3. You don't need to exercise in order to lose weight

   a. Exercise needs to be done in a gym

   b. Exercise needs to be done for at least 30 continuous minutes

4. If you buy it at a "health food" store or it's organic, then it's good for you (this seems obvious).

5. Muscle turns into fat (two totally different tissues in your body. Increasing muscle does however increases metabolism & makes the circumference of your limbs decrease = you look more toned).

6. Eating after 8 p.m. is bad for you (another obvious one).

7. Starting a diet with a FAD or crash diet is an effective way to lose weight (put me on the Cabbage Soup diet for a week & then I'll be ready to kill someone).

8. I'll never lose weight, it's in my genes

   a. I have a thyroid problem

   b. I have a slow metabolism

9. Natural or herbal weight-loss products are always safe and effective. (Arsenic is natural, but it can kill you.)

10. Fast foods are always unhealthy & you should never eat them. (There are always healthy options at your fingertips.)

11. Skipping meals is a good way to lose weight. (It actually makes your body think it's starving. Fire up your metabolism by eating more frequently throughout the day.)

12. Going vegetarian means you'll lose weight and be healthier. (In its true form, yes; however "vegetarian" something different to everyone. Most people are "crapatarians" who choose to not eat animal foods.)

You are what you eat!

Now that you've finished *Living Skinny in Fat Genes*™ don't tuck it away on a shelf. Keep it out so you can refer to it. Think of me as your wellness coach and that each day is a chance for you to live a healthy fulfilling life. Diet and exercise are the least expensive, least invasive and most effective ways to prevent and treat disease. So, what are you waiting for? Every day you can make choices in the foods and beverages that you consume and the physical activity you engage in . . . think about your goals and objectives so that you are on your way to a healthy way to lose weight and feel great. Wishing you much happiness, peace and good health!

–Felicia

AUTHOR'S BIOGRAPHY

FELICIA STOLER is a doctorally trained registered dietitian, exercise physiologist, TV personality and expert consultant in disease prevention, wellness and healthful living. Felicia is uniquely qualified with her extensive education, credentials and training to write about health and wellness. During her medical residency program at ABC News's Medical Unit in 2006, Felicia experienced writing and reporting on all medical topics. She knows that the media is a great way to reach more people in order to provide accurate, impartial and science-based information, and through her career has developed extensive media contacts.

Dr. Stoler was the host of the second season of TLC's groundbreaking series *Honey, We're Killing the Kids!*, which took aim at the unhealthy lifestyles of families across the country, in an effort to motivate them to make positive changes. Felicia's boundless energy, and friendly and approachable personality has been part of her charm. She has become a national speaker on the topic of healthful living and weight reduction. Dr. Stoler authored the Current Comment for the American College of Sports Medicine on childhood overweight and obesity.

Nearly fourteen years ago, while working at ABC News, Felicia wanted to make a career change, and someone suggested that she go to school for something that she was passionate about. So while working fulltime at ABC News, she attended graduate school at night. Not only did she complete a double masters degree in nutrition and applied physiology from Columbia University, but also her dietetic internship. Her desire to continue her education, while a working mother of two, has only enhanced Felicia's expertise, as has her doctoral work, completed at the University of Medicine and Dentistry of New Jersey, in the area of worksite wellness. She completed a residency at Rutgers University Athletics and ABC News Medical Unit in 2006. Felicia became Dr. Stoler in January 2008 and was recognized as a Fellow of the American College of Sports Medicine.

Felicia has appeared on CNN's *Showbiz Tonight*, the *Today* show, *Good Morning America*, *The Mike & Juliet Show*, *The Star Jones Show* (Court TV), News 12 New Jersey, NJN, and *Dateline NBC* (first weight-loss challenge), WB 11, ABC News *Inside the Newsroom*, and WCAU-TV NBC 10 Live! (Philadelphia), WABC-TV (NYC), WPBX-TV (Boston), WFXT (Boston), WTVJ (Miami), WPEC-TV (West Palm Beach), KING-TV (Seattle), KTXL-TV (Sacramento), KMAX-TV (Sacramento), KCRA-TV (Sacramento). Every month more are added to the list. Felicia had the highest-viewed Talk Back media videos for ABC News *Hopkins*. In addition, she was invited to be a "surprise" fitness presenter at the 2006 National Governors' Association winter meeting.

Felicia has been quoted/cited/published in ABCNews *Hopkins*, ABCNews.com, AOL Body, Asbury Park Press, *BusinessWeek Online*, Courier-Post, *Fitness* magazine, Food Arts, Greater Media Newspapers, Health, Home News Tribune, iVillage, *Ladies' Home Journal*, LivingIn Holmdel/Marlboro, Marlboro Matters, Men's Health, *Newark Star-Ledger*, Nickelodeon's Parents Connect, NJ Blitz, *NJ Monthly* magazine, *NY Daily News*, *NY Post*, *NY Runner*, *Outside*, Oxygen, *Philadelphia Daily News*, *Prevention*, *Runners World*, *SELF*, *Shape*, *TASTE* magazine, *Teen Vogue*, *The Arizona Republic*, the Drudge Report, *LA Times*, *The Lancet*, The News Transcript, *NY Times*, The NYC Marathon Magazine, The Wellness Advisor, The Rush Limbaugh Show, TimeOut NY, USA Today Weekend, *Washington Post*, WebMD, *Women's Day*, *Women's Golf*, and *Women's Health*. Felicia was recently a case study finalist for The Hot Mommas® Project (2008–2009) and was selected by a panel as one of the twelve top hot case studies that serve as role models for women and girls around the globe.

Felicia has been sought after by industry because of her talent for translating the science into consumer-friendly messages. Felicia has been on the Medical Advisory Board of GNC and has provided services for Milk PEP/National Dairy Council, Eli Lilly, Unilever, Cargill, Nesquik, the Florida Department of Citrus, Frito Lay, Kashi, and the list keeps growing.

Felicia has served in many professional associations as a volunteer and leader; along with volunteering in her community. She has been a mentor to many students, in addition to inspiring and helping to change the lives of hundreds, if not thousands, of people.

Felicia is passionate about health and wellness. A mother of two, Felicia understands the importance of a maintaining a healthy lifestyle for herself and her family, along with trying to be superwoman. Felicia resides in New Jersey.

NUTRITION AND HEALTH WEBSITES

exerciseismedicine.org/

fnic.nal.usda.gov/nal_display/index.php?info_center=4&tax_
level=1

healthymeals.nal.usda.gov/nal_display/index.php?info_
center=14&tax_level=1

my.clevelandclinic.org/health/default.aspx

www.acsm.org

www.aicr.org

www.americaonthemove.org/

www.calorieking.com/

www.cancer.org

www.cdc.gov

www.diabetes.org

www.eatright.org

www.fruitsandveggiesmorematters.gov/

www.health.gov/dietaryguidelines/

www.healthfinder.gov/

www.healthierus.gov/

www.heart.org

www.mayoclinic.com/

www.mypyramid.gov

www.nhlbi.nih.gov/

www.nlm.nih.gov/medlineplus/nutrition.html

www.nutrition.gov

www.shapeup.org/shape/steps.php

www.thera-bandacademy.com